SECRETS OF MOTIVATING YOURSELF TO WELLNESS

RUDY KACHMANN, M.D.

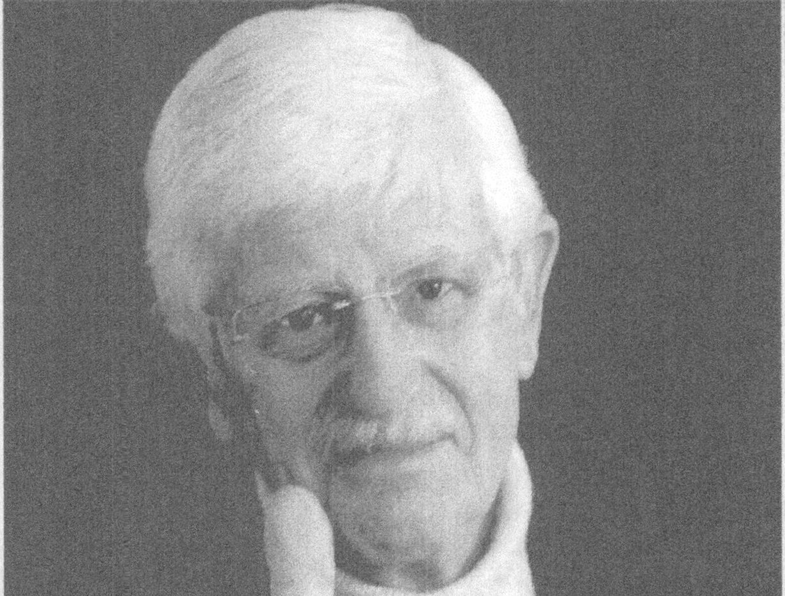

I'M YOUR COACH NOW

Published by Rudy Kachmann, M.D. Kachmann Media, LLC
www.KachmannMindBody.com

Library of Congress Control Number: 2010932480

ISBN-13: 978-1505585339

ISBN-10: 1505585333

Gary Ritter, Editor

Printed in the United States of America

TABLE OF CONTENTS

Recently, I was giving a lecture to a large group of medical providers about eliminating type 2 diabetes in 60 days, 90% of the time. I feel I can do that and it is supported in the literature with articles and books. One of the doctors in the audience stood up and said, "That's a very nice lecture, Dr. Kachmann, but how do I know or what are the odds of the patient doing what I asked them to do? How do I know what I said will motivate them? How do I know that on the way home, they will not stop at a fast food restaurant and continue on their merry way?"

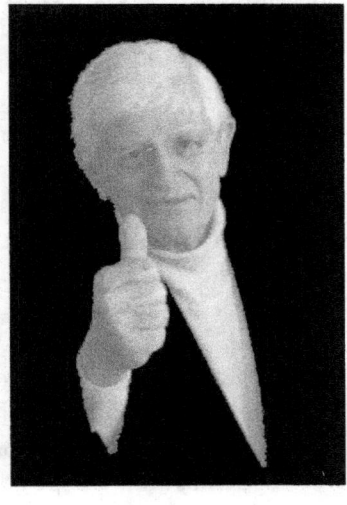

That raised a very important question in my mind. Because I believe what I teach, I think most audiences accept sincerely, what I say. I know that from many years of experience. But a good point is brought up here: do people stay motivated for a day, a week, a month or a lifetime? I suspect there are a great variety of responses. So how to motivate someone toward wellness became of great interest to me and resulted in this well-researched book.

My experience has taught me, as well as a research of the literature that there is a difference between motivating to success and motivating to wellness. Also, there are some things in common with motivating to success and wellness. Tamra Lowe, in her great book, Get Motivated, says that motivating toward success is in your genetic structure, it's in your genes or DNA. Matter of fact, she calls it motivational DNA. She says that there are about 82 things that might motivate a person toward success.

When I study the different cultures, societies, ethnic societies, I can see that the same races in different cultures have totally different incidences of diabetes, vascular disease and cancer. The China study proves that point. They studied one billion Chinese people and found it was their health habits and nutrition that determined their state of wellness. We see that also in the famous Pima Indian study in South America and Arizona. It is what you eat that determines the status of your health, not your genetic structure. It is my opinion that it is your family, culture and social surroundings and your personal choices that determine at least about 80% of your motivation toward wellness. I think it's about 40% family structure—their health habits—and about 40% personal choice. Perhaps about 20% is based on your genetic structure.

It is possible that we have what I call a "wellness gene," just like a thrifty gene for obesity, based on evolution. Some cultures, especially South American, African American and Micronesian have a thrifty gene that manifests itself. When they eat fat sugar and salt, they much more easily become overweight and develop diabetes. The Pima Indians in Arizona have a 90% diabetic rate. African-Americans in Africa have a low diabetes rate. But when they eat the mad sad American diet, the diabetes rate becomes high. I do wonder if we have "a wellness gene" that manifests itself with poor health habits.

Motivation is the power that creates action. It's like gas in your car and makes it move. Motivation is the fuel of success. All the health information in the world won't make you healthy unless you get moving. What can we do to motivate ourselves? How many things could motivate us to wellness? That is the subject of this book and you can see that there are many different ways.

Motivation to Wellness

There probably are as many ways of motivating someone, as there are people in the world. It probably takes a combination of 10 or so that will get the job done. But this combination is different for everyone, although you can certainly see that certain motivating things work better than others. Everyone is motivated differently. As Tamra Lowe said in her book, "There are probably no unmotivated people." Everyone is motivated, but they may be motivated to the wrong things. Motivated to sit on the couch and eat the wrong food, watch every sport contest that is on TV on the weekend, no exercise, and eating salt, sugar and fat all day long. Even criminals are motivated. What we need to do is to teach you how to motivate healthy activities, to live to be a hundred, mentally fit and physically fit, enjoying life every day along the way.

We all have our own unique motivational code. Which as you know, I think is a combination of genetic, family and personal choices. Each person has a unique psychological motivational pattern, and we have to discover what that is in you. It'll be a combination of drives, needs, and necessary rewards to stimulate you. It would be your wellness DNA that drives and rewards for doing the right thing. It will be different for each of us. You are made to be motivated in a specific way. Certain motivating things will excite and inspire you, and other motivators you will dislike and would never work with you.

Your enjoyment of life, the quality of your life, will be determined by your motivation. How long you live, how much disease will come to your life, how much you will enjoy life, will be determined by your motivation to wellness. The success or failure of relationships, finances, health, personal goals and general success in life will be determined by your motivation. We need to find out what your motivational DNA is.

I've put together about 39 motivational concepts that will help you. You will probably find that about 10 of them will work best for you, or maybe all of them. You certainly should read them all and then apply the best ones to yourself. You will have to make that decision. I do know and I am certain that you will have a more energetic life, happier life, live longer in good health, and have less disease, spend a lot less money on health care and spend less time in the hospital. This will get you to avoid drugs, injections, and unnecessary surgery, because you will be a much healthier individual. About 90% of the people in hospitals today are there because of poor lifestyle choices: poor eating habits, cigarettes, alcohol, and drug addictions. I want you to have a better life by motivating yourself toward wellness.

My recommendations work for everyone, no matter what gender, race or ethnic group, age, etc. What motivates one person may be de-motivating to another. So figure out your motivational DNA. You will be rewarded with good health.

Knowledge of the connection of Mind-Body-Spirit can be very motivating. Our body has a doctor living in it. It needs to be awakened; it knows how to get us well.

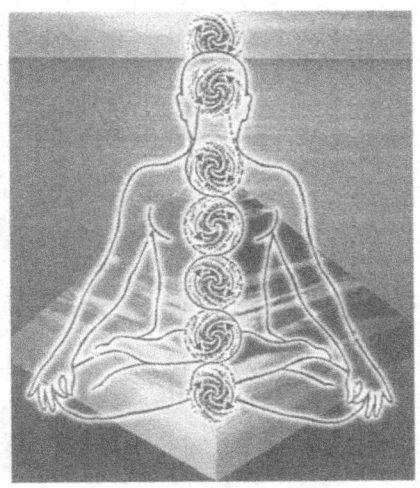

There's a connection of the mind with the body and the body with the mind. Dr. Candice Pert wrote a famous book called *Molecules of Emotion*. It explains the effects of your brain through neuropeptides (300 of them), hormones and neurotransmitters on your 60 trillion body cells. The 60 trillion body cells speak back to your body and brain with your eicosanoids, the Intel chips of your body made by every cell of your body. So how you think is everything. Your thought process leads the way.

No matter what your health problem is, how you think can have tremendous effects on these diseases and your well-being. Many can be cured by the proper practice of wellness, diet, exercise and positive thinking.

Many patients are not motivated to get better, some due to lack of knowledge of the mind-body connection, some due to the healthcare provider, who has no idea of the mind-body connection. That is, unfortunately, quite common. I know a number of cancer specialists who have no understanding whatsoever of the mind-body connection. The work of Dr. Carl Simonton, and Dr. La Shan has proven the benefits of mind-body techniques in the treatment of cancer. Studies have shown cancer patients can live twice as long if they practiced mind-body techniques, the spontaneous cure rate increases. The scientific proof goes back centuries.

The will to live has a commanding influence on motivation. Patients want their bodies fixed, but some don't want to be part of the team.

What Is Holistic Medicine?

You look at the physical aspect of the disease.
You look at the physiology of the disease.
You look to the spiritual aspect of the patient.
The patient must participate in the belief of their recovery.
The love of the family is important.
A placebo Dr. needs to be part of the team, as well as the patient.

What's Going on in Your Life?

Stress is a cause of numerous illnesses. I made a list of the illnesses caused by stress and put them in the "Mind Body Index", a name I copyrighted, just like a body mass index. I did that so that the public and the medical providers would pay more attention to illness caused by stress. We really don't find anything on any test. Yet, does a lot of operations on these patients unnecessarily, because they don't understand the concept of mind-body illness. Illness is the perception of being unwell. A partial list all of these illnesses are illustrated here:

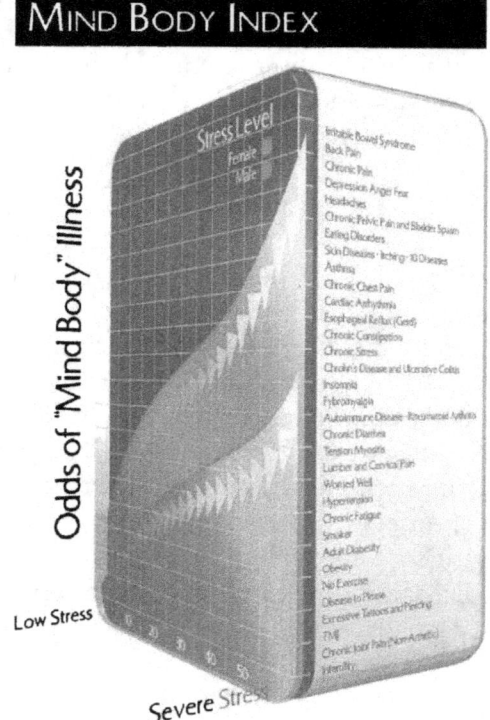

These illnesses can plague that patient, and they can spend a lifetime on them. Once a person has been educated to believe his or her illness is due to stress and the symptoms are real, then the healing can begin.

Education is the motivation factor in my experience. It may take some work. Some patients and families are just incredulous when I tell them it's a stress problem, nothing life-threatening is going on. They have been so fixated on an MRI report and believed their body was falling apart, when it's only the process of aging and nothing unusual. The over reading of CT scans, MRI's and angiograms is a serious problem, leading to a lot of unnecessary medical care. The interpretation of these studies and their relationship to the patient's symptoms are the critical factor. A lot of it depends whether you going to a placebo or a nocebo healthcare provider. Read my chapter on placebo for more details. A placebo doctor educates the patient with some material to read, recommends DVDs, CDs and meditation, which can motivate them to wellness. It may take a few visits to get the job done, but that is the job of the family physician to start. If the family physician is not a motivator or a placebo doctor, it's a real problem, because 50 to 75% of the patients need that. You can take the stress test associated with my mind-body index to judge the probability of you having or developing a mind-body disease.

The point is, if you can see the connection, if you have one of these mind-body illnesses, you can be cured. You can avoid a lot of unnecessary procedures by reading my book *Welcome to Your Mind-Body*. It explains what the mind-body connection is in detail. It can save you a lot of pain, unnecessary procedures, and a lot of money. If you don't have a mind-body disease, I guarantee you, your friends or relatives have one and maybe they have them all, as I've seen in some of my patients. My educating them has helped a great deal.

Fear and anxiety can reduce our motivation. Many die a thousand deaths. Most are suffering from the most common affliction, anxiety. Inability to cope with perceived or real threats to our physical, spiritual and emotional 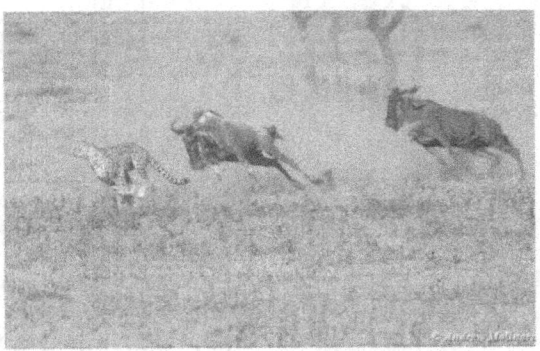 well being is the best definition of chronic long-term stress. It is accompanied many times by the next step up—depression. Depression reduces our motivation further. We want to sleep and hide. It may lead to a worse mental problem—schizophrenia. But we don't have to think. Schizophrenics readily rarely die from cancer—they don't get destructive stress—they live in a dream world. Lunatics live longer; they don't worry about anything. They don't get these destructive steroids that kill the Intel chips of our body, the eicosanoids. Anxiety and depression are destructive states. They rob us all of our motivation. Health is not a stable condition. For most, like a steel building or a concrete foundation, health is a state of balance maintained by personal adjustments, habits, from within and from out.

Anxiety is a sign that the will to live, which is motivating, is under direct attack. Depression is a step further; it indicates a partial surrender to death. Anxiety shows in the mind thoughts that all life is threatened.

We cannot always avoid anxiety, but we need not remain its defenseless victims. Rest and sleep recapture the body's energy. I have 20 prescriptions for stress reduction. My patients have found them to be very helpful. They are also on my Web site, *www.kachmannmindbody.com*. Medications may help depression and stress, but too many times they are not the final answer. The cause must come under control and be dealt with, if possible. Medicine generally is not the cure. The body may rebel and the stress then comes out as a mind-body illness. Health is not merely the absence of physical illness or disease. Emotional illness is an illness in its own right.

Anxiety is a whisper from the unconscious. Whether it's real or imagined, the threat to health is real. Depression is a partial surrender to death. A tranquil mind is a mind well ordered. Each man has within himself the power to destroy as well as preserve himself. A man in conflict is like a country in a civil war. There is a potential healing—or a good placebo doctor—or the doctor within us. Our body knows how to get well—we just have to do something to stimulate it.

Dr. Freud, a famous psychiatrist from Vienna at the beginning of the last century, came to the conclusion that we have only two basic psychological instincts, Eros and the destructive instinct. Eros, the god of love, is the creativity instinct. The intellectual and scientific and ceaseless struggle to advance oneself and to improve the world offered the expression of one compelling instinct, force, the creativity instinct. Many of us have it, some unfortunately don't. It is the will to live and to nurture life in all its varied forms.

The destructive instinct is a new and difficult concept. Freud called it the death instinct. I do wonder sometimes, when I see some of my patients on multiple narcotics with absolutely no interest in trying another way. I asked them why they're taking these medications, and the answer is, "I hurt." End of story. They get up and leave, having no interest in getting well. Clearly, a destructive impulse leading to big trouble, including the possibility of death. Ninety patients died in our surrounding counties this year from physician-written narcotic prescriptions. You think we have a problem? It's all over the nation.

It is that smoldering erosion force within us, which aims to directly and willfully destroy us. I agree with Dr. Freud; I cannot think of any other explanation. This mother of four children, no husband, under a great deal of stress, had no interest whatsoever to get the killing narcotics. It must be the chemical dopamine that's making it feel so good that she would never consider another alternative to an addictive life. It is nature's instrument to end life. This nation is on a very destructive path, and I'm sorry to say I could not think of anything that would motivate her. I think she could face death and still would take those drugs. Very unfortunate. The destructive force gains momentum and the creative powers in an individual are exhausted.

Freud also called it attraction and repulsion, which rule the inorganic world—fusion and fission, friendship and strife, love and hate. Good and evil, the concert is the same. The Chinese for 5000 years called it the yin and the yang. Opposites of the same hill, a blending of good and evil, not direct opposites. It's in the inner world of Everyman. Man turns the creative and destructive process upon himself. It is always painful to awaken to self-deception when a reality arrives, especially if the reality has no escape.

The mind pushes the stress below the level of consciousness, where we no longer feel its pain. Tiredness without exertion is a sign that energy's being used up, and not in a struggle between self-destruction and escape. People who are at odds with themselves, have little margin of safety and are ready victims of illness at critical times. The husband dies, and the wife dies from cancer within a year. That horrible stress, including others, reduces the will to live. It has been statistically shown that heart attacks, cancer and a number of other diseases follow high stress levels. The will to live dissipates. We pick our time of illness, and what type of illness, psychologically. Under stress, the mind gives warning signs to be heeded to those who wish to live in health. We ourselves choose a time of illness, the kind of illness, and its seriousness. How we think motivates our brain's brain, our Wizard of Oz, our metabolic control center, the hypothalamus to heal or destroy us. Our will to live can determine that.

The decision to create or to destroy us, made in the unconscious court of judgment, is influenced by our thought process. We may need mind-body illnesses to live, to avoid depression and suicide. The choice of a target organ for an illness is relegated to the unconscious ways of emotional experiences—an emotional need and a significant event to determine the time of illness. Many patients I treat have many of the illnesses on the mind-body index. I saw a young girl recently whose mother and brother had fibromyalgia. When I showed her the mind-body index in my book, she said, "I have them all." And after speaking to her for quite some time, I agreed. The mother and her two children had a number of mind-body illnesses due to stress in the family. Illness may come as a needed respite from problems we feel unable to solve, perhaps unable to face.

Illness may be an unconscious device to change a situation by influencing our and others' attitudes or behaviors toward us. Illness may be way to fight hostility, what we cannot accept within ourselves. And many illnesses may be acute, a way of getting out of a temporarily difficult situation. Or it may become chronic if the situation continues to be unresolved. Understanding of the deeper reasons promises a better way to deal with life situations, and also to safeguard our health. The will to live is critical for survival.

We must balance the books to have a healthy body. We must resolve our problems if possible. Practice stress-reduction techniques, as recommended in my 20 prescriptions on page x. The will to live can be strengthened, nourished, cultivated, and this can be done consciously. The patient has to become an active ally of the doctor. Often the patient has feelings of hostility, fear, and defensive obstinacy toward a doctor. Recognition of these feelings by the doctor enables the patient to cooperate with the doctor. The stress must be recognized by the physician and explained to the patient. Warning signals are fatigue, anxiety, hopelessness, guilt. They must be recognized by both parties. We must realize that stress is part of living, and it is necessary to deal with it. We must learn the measures to meet stress and break the tension and conserve and replenish our own energy. A good night's sleep is a great start, and we must work on that. Stress affects every aspect of the living, food, social activities, recreation, sleep, all have to be adjusted to the needs of the stressful.

A regimen for stress is different for each individual in each situation, but the goals are the same, to reduce tension and keep up energy. Exercise is very important all on a regular basis. I highly recommend taking short periods of time through the day for relaxation. I called them "a pause in time", and do something totally different from work for about10 minutes three times a day. I sit at a coffee shop reading a book or writing my books, something totally different from neurosurgery. I find it very relaxing. To allow cells to become run down on stress is self-destructive. To learn meditation is very helpful. Get involved with music. Norman Cousins wrote that famous book, *Getting Well Again*; I suggest you read it. My book, *Welcome to Mind-Body*, will tell you the science behind mind-body illnesses, their cause and their treatment.

Living is an art in which everyone begins as an amateur. The experience of others, or escape into fantasy and drugs and wishful thinking are make-believe living. It will lead to the loss of the will to live. There is a doctor living within all of us. We can stimulate the will to live. Live in the present moment—we can't change the past—and work on the future.

We need to cultivate the will to live. The enjoyment of both work and play is a symptom of a flourishing will to live. Personally, I work very hard at age 74, in full-time neurosurgery, trade my own stocks, practice music every morning, read and write books in the morning, start surgery at 9:30, play tennis at night, and give at least one lecture a week. I feel great almost everyday. Incidentally, I follow a flexitarian diet, as recommended in my book, *The Secret of the Nondiet*. I'm just advising, not bragging. If I didn't do it, how could I teach it? Aging is relevant to me. Many grow old before they grow up. Staying young means keeping up the active interests of youth. The mind, like muscles, goes flabby with disuse. An active and interested mind never grows old! The measure of man's life is not the length but the quality.

"You cannot teach a man anything, you can only help him to find it within himself." —Galileo. Doctors in the past have been the first healers, then scientists. The doctor of the future is both scientist and healer. I'm sorry to say, that is not happening very much today. The true meaning of doctor is teacher. His job is not only to cure, but to teach patients how to be well. Amen.

See Dr. Kachmann's 20 Daily Prescriptions To Reduce Stress On Next Page

Dr. Kachmann's 20 DAILY PRESCRIPTIONS TO REDUCE STRESS

1. CREATE A SPIRITUAL, SAFE PLACE IN THE HOME
    a. Three minutes of abdominal breathing that is calm and focused

2. MEDITATE
    a. Concentrate on you nasal breath.
    b. Next concentrate on you abdomen going up and down.
    c. Say or chant a mantra (mind energy) multiple times. For example-Spirit, God, Om, Sat Nam, Let Go, Be Free, I'm Happy,etc.

3. VISUALIZE AN IMAGE DAILY OF WHAT YOU WANT TO ACHIEVE THAT DAY OR IN THE FUTURE

4. SAY SOMETHING THANKFUL WHEN YOU GO TO BED EVERY NIGHT AND SAY SOMETHING OPTIMISTIC OR JOYFUL EVERY MORNING

5. MANAGE YOUR FINANCES WELL BECAUSE IT IS ONE OF THE BIGGEST CAUSES OF STRESS
    a. Get your finances organized.
    b. Don't panic and remember to breathe.
    c. Be disciplined and know your debts.
    d. Make a new plan by thinking your way out of it and seeing a new way of making it.

6. DON'T FOCUS ON NEGATIVITY
    a. Avoid T.V., radio, and bad news media. Media Fast.
    b. Don't spend the whole night on the computer or watching TV, give yourself time to transition into sleep, read a book, relax let the mind unwind.
    c. News/media are preoccupied with gloom and doom, crime, world pain, murder, mayhem and perversion, give it a rest.

7. PRACTICE YOGA, TAI CHI, WALKING, DANCING, OR ENJOY EXERCISES THAT BRING ABOUT RELAXATION AND

MEDITATION RATHER THAN OVERSTRESSING THE BODY
AND MIND

8. EACH DAY SPEND 15-30 MINUTES PRACTICING
MEDITATIVE WALKING. "WALKING MEDITATION"
   a. Use your senses explore the present moment.
   b. Appreciate sounds, appreciate what you see, and appreciate
   nature

9. THINK POSITIVELY
   a. Be hard-headed and tough-minded, refuse to let others bring
   you down.
   b. Don't give up believe in yourself.
   c. Make a plan to solve the problem.
   d. Write a plan and visualize it daily.

10. LIVE IN THE PRESENT MOMENT NOT IN THE FUTURE
OR PAST
   a. Live in the light of the day not in the storm of yesterday and
   tsunami of tomorrow.

11. ENJOY MUSIC IN YOUR HOME AND IN YOUR CAR ON
THE WAY TO WORK AND BACK
   a. It is the language of God or Spirit.
   b. Music sound is medicine. It is the bridge between spirit and
   matter.

12. EAT PROPER FOOD
   a. Food is a drug don't abuse it.
   b. Don't use food to manage your psychology because it is not a
   good stress reducer.
   c. Read the Secret of the Non-Diet. It is about proper food
   selection.

13. ORGANIZE YOUR TIME
   a. Demand at least 15-30 minutes for your self daily, no matter
   what the situation is.

14. TREAT YOURSELF TO A MASSAGE LET GO OF THE MONKEY MIND
    a. Take a mind shampoo and clean your mind of stress daily. How you think is everything.

15. DON'T SMOKE, USE ILLEGAL DRUGS, OR EXCESSIVE MEDICATIONS
    a. In the long run, they will cause stress.

16. FALL IN LOVE WITH YOURSELF AND APPRECIATE THE LOVE OF THE FAMILY NO MATTER WHAT THE PROBLEMS ARE

17. BE A HAPPY PERSON
    a. Avoid negative thoughts or statements. No one can solve all the worlds' problems, so don't focus on them.

18. LIVE THE LIFE OF GRATITUDE RATHER THAN A LIFE OF REGRET.
    a. You can't change the past.
    b. Say nice things to people all day like "You look great" "Have a nice day" or "Thank you again".

19. LET GO OF SELF JUDGMENT AND SELF CRITICISM
    a. You are the creation of spirit or God. He does not make mistakes.

20. KNOW WHAT MIND-BODY ILLNESSES OR STRESS RELATED ILLNESSES ARE
    a. Stress causes 75% of the illnesses that we see a doctor about. Wellness and stress education is what you need 75% of the time.
    b. Avoid unnecessary tests and procedures
    c. By understanding what the illnesses are, I have gathered them together in the Mind Body Index.
    d. Read *Welcome to your Mind Body*. It will save you money in medical care, reduce your stress, and cure your problems with the proper techniques as recommended above.

A Sense of Purpose

How can we continue doing the same thing and expect a different outcome?

We all want a better life, better health, financial gains, determination to beat that serious illness, and a whole host of other things that we anticipate will give us that sense of

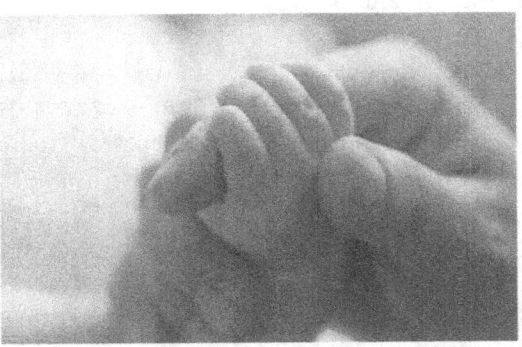

purpose we so desire. How can we accomplish these huge goals? What will get us progressing in the right direction?

As a wellness doctor and lecturer, I give both patient and audience the education and the scientific background to stimulate change by teaching the wellness aspect of illness and disease. But is that really enough to get the job done? How motivating am I? Do my words lead to short-term or long-term changes in my listeners? I've certainly seen changes in my patients; some short-term and others long-term, and yet I suspect some others do not change at all. I practice what I preach and I presume that to be motivating. And so I aim for long-term changes in my patients.

Correlation is used to urge interaction, but it may be short-term. What you need is change that endures. You must be proactive if you plan to change your life. Changes need to be started immediately or the commitment will leave you. Consistency in what you are doing can leave quickly as feelings interfere. Now you have another failed attempt, and you feel discouraged. A shaky commitment can get in the way of purposeful motivation.

Creating a sense of purpose for your life and doing something to duplicate that is more likely to result in a permanent change and accomplish your goal.

When you set out to create and accomplish, while stimulated by this sense of purpose, you are most likely to cause these long-term changes within yourself.

Motivation solves short-term problems, but for long-term results, you must find the root of your sense of purpose and renovate it. When we are fearful, we go for quick fixes. Drugs, cigarettes, and food are all chemicals that affect the mind for a quick fix. And of course that only leads to more problems - poor health, family conflict, job loss...the list goes on and on.

If you were to develop a sense of purpose in life, you are most likely to reach your long-term goal, and your subconscious mind will help you to get there. The famous cancer psychotherapist Dr. Lawrence LeShan found during 45 years of treating cancer patients that if he could find or discover a purpose in life for his cancer patient, he could double his or her lifespan and increase the likelihood of a spontaneous cure of the cancer. A sense of purpose stimulates activity in the immune system, improving both longevity and cure rate.

Now sit down with a pencil and paper and write down what you are trying to accomplish, whether it be weight loss, transforming your appearance, improving family relations, a career change, or getting rid of bad habits such as smoking and/or drinking. If you establish a sense of purpose to improve yourself, it is much more likely you will reach your goal and make it happen.

For example, although I am in my early 70s, I have created a sense of purpose by planning to be the national 80-and-over tennis champ. I am already training for it. I take a tennis lesson once a week from the best player in town, do yoga and weight training three days a week, and play tennis at night on a regular basis. It has given me a reason to get out of bed and I have a sense of great purpose. This is what motivates me.

Additionally, I am writing books, creating DVDs, giving a great number of lectures on wellness, and practicing neurosurgery full-time. At 73, I have developed a sense of purpose that is very motivating. I wake early at 5:00 a.m. and start my day reading, writing, working out, and practicing my saxophone. By nine o'clock, I take a pause at Starbucks to meet friends and get ready for the day's work. I can't say it enough: I feel a great sense of purpose in helping others get well. I hope you can find your purpose in life. It will motivate you to get the job done.

Look for a sense of purpose, like getting in shape. For example, type 2 diabetes is curable in 30 days by eating the right foods. Or, improve the relationships within your family. If you have self-induced physical problems, eliminate them. If you die, think of this - it is your family that will cause to suffer.

You need to find your song, the one that makes you move permanently in the direction of your goals and gives vision to your life.

We all have a unique song to sing no matter what the circumstance. Find your unique individual music and make it positive! It will improve your self-image and it will be a call to action. All people have a natural way of relating and creating, and when you find yours, you will fulfill your dreams.

You need to take control over your own life; no one will do it for you. "I just can't do it" are not acceptable words. Visualize a life you would like to live and work towards it every day, even if you are only making small changes. The changes will stimulate your immune system and your subconscious mind, and visualizing it will make it much more likely to happen. We can keep on doing the same things and expect different results, but that is just insanity.

When you have discovered your purpose, immediately begin to create momentum. Write down your purpose or goal frequently, and then do something daily to work toward this goal with some positive action. Set a three month, six month, and one-year goal, and have a little celebration when you achieve these goals.

Helping others may be the most motivating thing you can do; it sure works for me. Spirituality and religion create purpose for many people. Senseful purpose is the food on which our souls can thrive.

Your age does not matter—use me as an example. We all need something to strive toward, so we can design our own inspiration. This will be different for different people. The secret to living is to create a meaningful purpose. The first step to creating any change is to make the decision of what you want, not what you don't want. That is what will create a purpose in your life. Twenty percent of change is to know how to create it; and if you have opposition to change you need to know why you're doing it.

Dr. Rick Warren, famous evangelist, affirms that purpose is not a list of goals. Goals are temporary; purposes are eternal. It is a statement that points the direction of your life. He would say that if you tie your direction to your spiritual leader, whether that be God, Mohamed, or Jesus, it is much more likely to happen. Writing down your purposes forces you to think specifically about the path of your life, and knowing which way you are headed will keep you on solid ground. An intelligent person knows the direction he is going, but a fool starts going off in many different directions. Find out what your purpose is and start working on it today.

As a physician, I consider myself to be a teacher; after all, that is what the word means. So I have a built-in desire to make people well. Frankly, I like to be called Dr. Wellness. The mayor of our city called me that at a recent meeting. And I am proud of that.

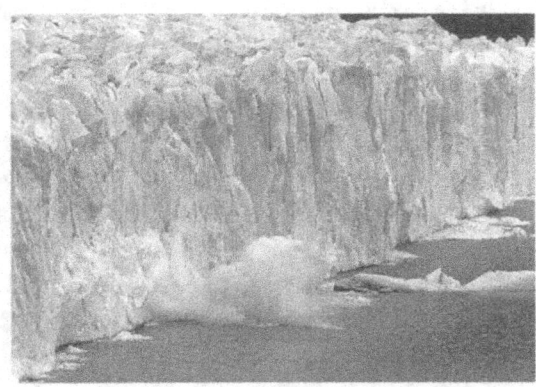

Being a physician, of course, I see patients every day who need wellness teaching. They wouldn't come to see me if they had no problems. But how do you facilitate change? How do you motivate someone toward wellness? I do take the time, maybe even 30 minutes, to educate the patient toward wellness. It's a noble desire to change someone; it's actually my job. We may certainly differ in what the right path is. Motivation is an interpersonal process—an interaction between two people. Motivation for change cannot only be influenced by us, but in a very real sense, arises from an interpersonal context. We may assume that the person is already motivated for change when he comes to see us, but most of the time that is not true. Many want a quick fix, a pill, a procedure, or maybe even an operation, which may not be needed. I see that all the time. Exploring and enhancing motivation for change is a necessary task for us and our physician, if we plan to get well.

Many times, the person you're trying to change, including yourself, is ambivalent about the need of it. The patient should be voicing the arguments for change, or you yourself may express these opinions and feel the need of it. But that is not always the case. If you or the patient is voicing arguments against change, I have to be very careful as to what I say, or I will never convince you to do it. Both parties often leave the interaction frustrated and dissatisfied, each blaming the other, and very little positive change occurs. I have had it happen to me more than once, tried to convince a patient to follow a certain course of wellness instead of having injections or operations or using narcotics for their non-specific pain. Motivational interviewing is more like dancing, while rather than struggling against each other, you have to move together smoothly, but nothing will happen. Motivating change needs imagination.

You have to develop and point out a discrepancy in the other person's interpretation of the present state of health. How they think and what actual reality is. You may think you look good being overweight, but you're not looking at what's going to occur in the future. You're not looking at what is going on inside your body: diabetes, arthritis, heart disease, etc. The discrepancy is generally between the present status and a desired goal of good health. The difference between what is happening and how we would like things to be—to be healthy, look good, and live a long life. The larger the discrepancy, the greater the importance of change.

Because it involves perception, however, discrepancy is more complex than just noticing the difference between what is and what should be. One's behavior can come into conflict with a deeply held value without there being a change in either. As I've heard many times: although I have heart disease and diabetes, I can't give up eating meat. This happens particularly when there is a change, not in the behavior, but in the perceived meaning of the behavior. When a behavior comes into conflict with a deeply held value, it is usually the behavior that changes. So it is very important to know what the deeply held values are. That might motivate us to change. For example to stop smoking, so the children don't become sick. For some people, the first step toward change becomes ambivalent. As discrepancy increases, ambivalence first intensifies; then if the discrepancy continues to grow, ambivalence can be resolved in the direction of change. Ambivalence is not really an obstacle to change; it is what makes change possible.

So the challenge is to first to identify and then resolve ambivalence by developing discrepancy between the actual present situation and the desired future. It can be very difficult. When I'm speaking to patients to change them in a 30 minute interview, a number of them completely agree while in front of me and even express a desire to change, man and wife may both agree, but nothing happens. Others go to my Wellness Center and buy my books and DVDs and continue their education to change. Follow-up appointments are very important so that I can re-motivate the patient. I encourage them to attend my lectures, which are free, for further education. Of course, attending the lectures is a sign of motivation, and many times does induce change.

Change is facilitated by communicating in a way that elicits a person's own reasons for an advantage of change. I examined a patient like that yesterday and took full advantage of his pointing out the discrepancy between his behaviors in what was going on. He was killing himself from type 2 diabetes.

I pointed out to him the disadvantages of the status quo. I pointed out to him the advantages of change. I prayed for his optimism to change, that he could get the job done and he expressed an intention to change. I tried to get him to commit to change in front of his wife. To get someone else involved with the commitment increases the chances of that actually happening.

Motivating Happiness

Your brain makes hormones, neurotransmitters, and neuropeptides that make you feel good. The main chemicals are dopamine, serotonin and noradrenalin. They can motivate you into good or bad habits. Food breaks down into feel-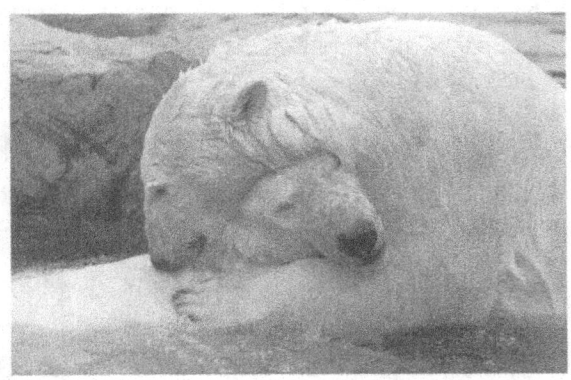good chemicals. You can use food to make yourself feel good and a lot of people do, so you have to be careful. You have to know the difference. Drug abusers like the feeling created by the chemical dopamine...but there isn't any feeling you can get on drugs that you can't get without drugs.

Make a commitment to yourself to find the natural highs. You need to stay motivated. For example, exercise will cause the secretion of endorphins, your own safe morphine that makes you feel good. You can stimulate these brain chemicals by activating them through laughter, singing, dancing, exercising, or hugging someone. When you're having fun, your body chemistry changes. You can get new biochemical surges of motivation and energy.

A recent patient I saw was taking morphine every day for headaches and neck pain of unclear cause. She was divorced and the mother of four children. It was chemicals in the narcotics, dopamine, serotonin that gave her such a good feeling. She was unwilling to give up them no matter what. Believe me, I tried. She just walked out of the room and didn't want to listen to what she was doing to herself. I think she already was an addict, created by physician prescriptions, which I see very commonly. She could've gotten the same high from exercise, laughter, and stress-reduction techniques. She was on the road to nowhere, perhaps even jail.

Once you've made it past pain, you solve the problem of self-motivation by trying to go outside yourself searching for something that's fun. It's not out there anywhere; it's inside you. The opportunity for fun is in your own energy system, your synergy of heart and mind. That's where you will find it. If your activity is not fun, you're not doing it right. For example, I make a consistent effort to find humor when dealing with my patients. Under the most trying circumstances, even discussions of life and death, generally I can find something to put a smile on myself and the other person. A simple hug at the end of a conversation always makes me feel good and at times when I'm on the elevator at the hospital, where most visitors have a concern about something, I try to make a funny remark. And in spite of everything, they generally laugh.

Norman Cousins, author of the book, *Anatomy of an Illness*, found that watching funny movies relieved his pain for many hours. It was feel-good chemicals called endorphins, serotonin, dopamine and noradrenalin. Don't produce a feeling with dangerous drugs; you can produce them through normal activities. That's just as good, much healthier, and very motivating. A natural high brings a lot more happiness than a drug-induced high. Once we have a great feeling from natural activities, like exercise, laughter and family, it becomes addictive.

MOTIVATION OF FOOD

The main road to wellness is driven by eating the correct food. If you want to live to be a hundred and be mentally sound, eating the right food, exercising, stress control, and a purpose in life is what you need.

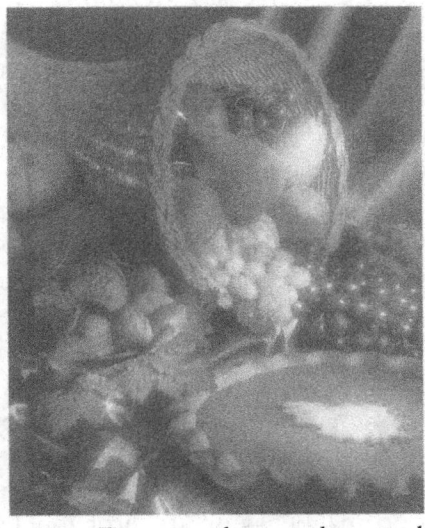

Fat, sugar, and salt are being used by the food industry to kill us. It's the cause of 90% of the illnesses and diseases that I, as a doctor, see every day. Being a neurosurgeon, 80% of the patients I see have a back problem. The causes are lack of exercise and being overweight, the majority of the time. Everyone has an abnormal MRI of the spine and the amount of injections and operations I see is beyond description. Everyone has screws and rods in their back—instead of weight loss and exercise.

What motivates us to eat the wrong food, and then, to top it all off, too much of it? You don't see that in a lot of the world, China, Japan, Asia, and some parts of Africa. Although, it's starting to change.

The causes are numerous. We live in the highly stressful West; bad food is cheap; we have no time to fix a healthy meal; our knowledge of proper eating is limited. Doctors don't even know what to tell you themselves. We use food to treat our anxiety and depression. Fatty and sugary foods motivate us to get serotonin—a chemical to make us feel better— a cheap prescription.

Food is a drug, just like nicotine, alcohol, cocaine. It reduces our pain. A nonprescription drug to make us feel better. Food has tremendous motivational power. The psychological aspect is very complex.

We can eat too much or too little. Patients with anorexia nervosa are motivated to thinness and refuse to eat. They look in the mirror and, although very thin, they see a fat person, a mistaken perception. Just like a heavyset person can look in the mirror and see a normal person, they do not see themselves as they actually are. The majority of us, when we have a stressful day, are motivated to grab the first thing out of the refrigerator or stop at a fast food restaurant and eat something nasty with a lot of fat, sugar and salt. It's because we are stressed and treating our mind with serotonin. We need a quick fix.

The visualization or sight of the food, the Golden Arches, is the cue that releases dopamine from the hypothalamus in our brain. Food releases serotonin and endorphins to make us feel good and reduce our stress level. Some foods metabolize into beta-endorphin and dynorthin, which not only make us feel good, but also stimulate eating behavior. Dynorphin causes a ravenous appetite. A very obese person most likely operates on a lot of dynothin. I normally watch what I eat very carefully, but last Tuesday I worked all day and was on call all night long for neurosurgery for the whole area. I did two major brain operations for trauma and then worked the next day doing three elective surgeries. Frankly, I grabbed a piece of lousy food in the doctors' lounge between operations and felt I had a license to do it. A total breakdown of my normal behavior, and probably I was operating on beta-endorphin and dynorpin. I felt helpless to my impulses.

If you need one doughnut and can't help yourself, you probably have been motivated by a team of endorphins. One potato chip, and away we go. The chemicals of food, you can see, are very motivating to overeating and lead to poor health, sedentary behavior, and obesity.

The main culprits are fat, sugar and salt, the children of fast food restaurants. If you eat high-nutrient-dense food, not calorie-dense food, like refined foods stripped of their nutrients, you will not be exposed to many of these stimulating food chemicals. You can get over sugar addiction in 21 days. You can get over a fat addiction in 21 days. The phytochemicals in nutrient-dense foods will turn your appetite down and you will feel full, and much healthier. Read my book, The Secret of the Non-diet, avoid the mad, sad, toxic American diet that is killing us. America has the highest rate of diabetes and vascular disease in the world, as well as cancer.

It is the chemicals that cause psychological changes in the body and motivate us to disease and illness. Motivate yourself by understanding clearly that the mad, sad, toxic American way of eating leads to many diseases and will cut your life short. Besides, you won't feel very good, and probably won't look very good. The China study by Dr. Colin Campbell of the diets and diseases of one billion Chinese people proved that what we eat is directly related to the diseases and illnesses we develop. The communities who ate a high nutrient way of eating, vegetarian, vegan, flexitarian, high-nutrient-dense types of food had very little illness. Probably eating will motivate you to good health,

LIFE CHANGING EVENTS

A life-altering event can be very motivating for short-term and especially long-term changes. It can bring the inspiration to get the job done.

Since it was close to New Year's Eve when I was fired from my job at 7 p.m. in 1969, my story comes to mind first. I remember the story like it happened yesterday. It caused me so much stress in my life.

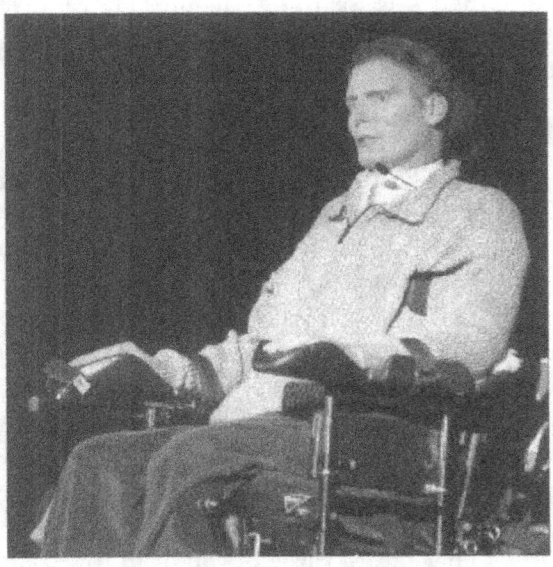

I had started my neurosurgery practice on July 1, 1969 in association with one other neurosurgeon in Fort Wayne, Indiana. I had just completed my neurosurgery training at Georgetown University and a two-year stint with the US Navy and Marines during the Vietnam War.

I thought my partner and I got along fairly well and had no unusual problems or arguments. We were so busy we never even took weekends off.

On New Year's Eve, December of 1969 about 6 p.m. my partner called and asked if he could come over. I assumed it was to give me a bonus. My wife and I were getting dressed to go to a New Year's Eve party. He rang the doorbell, and there he stood with an envelope in one hand and a box in the other. The box was not gift wrapped, but I thought it was a present, anyway. I opened the envelope, and instead of having a check for my family, it was a letter stating that he was terminating our partnership, as of midnight. Then he changed the locks on the office and the locks of the closet with the surgical instruments, essentially putting me totally out of business—and the practice of medicine.

It was devastating to my family and me. I had a wife and three little children, a home and a lake cottage, two mortgages, $50,000 in school debts, plus about $10,000 in credit card debts. Up till then I had a good salary and a bright future. I had good results from surgeries without any serious complications. He didn't even give me a month's wages so I could get myself on my feet and find another job. He clearly had planned this for quite a while. He then sued me for about $20,000, because I had accepted insurance as payment in full from a number of patients who had no money, a usual thing a reasonable doctor does. He said I had no authority to do that since he owned the practice. To this day I have never really understood why he did that.

I spoke to a patient yesterday, and we were discussing stressful times. I was trying to give an example to make him feel better, because he lost his job. He said, "You know, Doctor, it's all about money." I suspect he may be right. Unfortunately.

This was my first Christmas out of many years of school. So you can see why I overspent. My kids normally didn't have much of a Christmas.

What do you think? Was this a motivating event? Of course, I was seriously distressed, couldn't sleep for six weeks, but I did not completely panic.

I did some hard thinking, made a plan. I had no office, no instruments, and no patients.

There were three hospitals in town, but none of the surgeons had their office next to the Lutheran Hospital, a fairly large, high-quality hospital. So I set up an office 100 feet from the emergency room, sharing the office of a generous physician. He let me use the office rent-free for a few months. I remember the day he offered that space to me like it was yesterday. There also was a well-known clinic next door, which I joined immediately; this gave me some referrals, which helped put food on the table for my family. I was also close to the emergency room; this allowed me to see the majority of patients I also made myself available around the clock.

What's the lesson? Think hard and then do something. Sitting around and doing nothing will produce nothing. You'll retire on an unemployment check, or with an overweight or obesity problem, do something about your situation now so this does not happen to you. It was very motivating to have debts, no money and a wife and three children. And two parents who couldn't work anymore and who had no money in their bank account either. The city at that time had some very excellent neurosurgeons, come to find out, not all were nice people, and so competition was stiff. So I did some more hard thinking. It turned out my next project affected all of the city of Fort Wayne to this day. I opened clinics in four small rural Ohio hospitals. I would go there and see the patients and if they needed surgery, I would do it in Fort Wayne. I was very busy and so was Fort Wayne. Doctors in other specialties copied what I did.

Eventually, I went to four small hospitals on the same day. I'd get home at 10 p.m. or so, No one ever had done that in Fort Wayne, and now all major specialty groups do it that is why Ft. Wayne is now a high-specialty-referral center. We now cover about a million people in the surrounding areas.

I could have left town like my partner suggested. Instead I made a plan. I visualized the goal to form a large neurology, neurosurgery referral group. Guess what? It happened. Of course, other people have different circumstances. Economic threat can become very motivating. Don't panic; deal with the stress, and think hard and do something. Turns out, it was actually God sent and accounts for a great deal of my success. Don't take revenge, the other guy's out dancing while you're planning it. Success speaks for itself.

If you have health issues with obesity, diabetes, or vascular disease, think out a plan to do something about it. The majority of illnesses I see are self-induced. Weight loss and exercise would cure the majority of them. When the potential side effects are a product of what you're eating, smoking, drinking, or using as drugs, then do something about it. You will look better, feel better, and live longer. Take a realistic look in the mirror and see the future and do something about it. About six times last year I was seeing patients who thought they were pregnant and that was the cause of their back pain. Turns out it was nothing but fat. I showed them the CT scan of the abdomen without the baby and that pointed out the fat. That was motivating to a lot of them. I actually had to run a pregnancy test to prove it to them. Many are able to ignore the belly hanging down, but I tell you, the fat in the abdomen has many nasty chemicals in it, causing major vascular disease, Alzheimer's disease, and cancer. If you want to significantly increase your risk of a heart attack at a young age, carry a big abdomen. Knowing what might happen is motivating to some people, but not everyone.

I suspect one issue is: if you think you're pregnant and you're not. I have seen that being motivating for certain people also. If you go to your doctor and he says you have type 2 diabetes, I have great news for you. If you return your weight to a normal BMI, Body Mass Index, you have a 90% chance of getting rid of and being cured of your type 2 diabetes. I know it works because I run wellness eating classes all the time and have cured many patients of type 2 diabetes and that is just fantastic news. And I love to talk about it. It's like getting a monkey off your back. If someone in your family has died of a heart attack at a young age, or has a stroke, check your weight and your blood. If either one is abnormal, try eating that proper diet. If that doesn't work, you may need medication so the same thing doesn't happen to you.

It can become more difficult to motivate yourself if you're on medication, but only you can make the decision. The same goes for alcohol and cigarettes. Seeing your friends or someone in the family dying from these conditions, losing their job, or breaking up families is motivating for some people, but not the majority. Sometimes it takes counseling and group therapy. I have seen some people that made up their mind and started doing these things, they became very healthy and that was the end of their problem. Working with groups, friends or relatives can be very helpful also.

Of course, since I treat a lot of serious spinal injuries, I've seen a lot of paraplegia and quadriplegia. In spite of these serious conditions, I've had a number of them become extremely successful. It looked like the injuries inspired them. I met a quadriplegic one time at the swimming pool at my condominium in Florida, just so happens he invented Post-it notes. He also owned a lot of printing companies, and I guess he was a billionaire. He felt being paralyzed inspired him, a great story. "I run wheel chair tennis tournaments at Indiana University and Purdue University every year, as well as support wheel chair basketball. These people despite their handicaps are great athletes. Injuries or disabilities can be inspiring and motivating. It really depends on what happens to you.

The story of Helen Keller is a classic example of motivation. In spite of being blind and deaf, she achieved great things, from writing poetry to constantly inspiring other people. She was motivated by her disabilities.

My last story is from my friend Jack, whom I met at Starbucks while reading a book. In December 2004, he stated, his life was a wreck. He was diagnosed with type 2 diabetes, weighed 265 pounds, had a blood pressure of 204/154; his marriage was on the rocks; his career was in a shambles. He was almost bankrupt, had $102,000 in credit card debt, hated everyone and everything, and it was God's fault.

One day while driving on the freeway to work, feeling really low, he looked up at the sky and yelled at God," Where the hell are you? I've done all the things I'm supposed to do and where are you? Why aren't you helping me? Why are you allowing all this crap to happen to me? He was blaming everyone and everything except the person truly responsible for his mess—himself. He had read scripture. He could even quote those verses one could use to explain his mediocrity. He went to church regularly, had been saved, knew how to pray, did all the things that good Christians do, but he had never really believed nor did he internalize the real meanings of these activities—like accept responsibility for his own life.

He dressed the part, long-sleeved white shirts, button-down collars, appropriate color tie, dark suit and shined shoes. He played the part, good guy, good husband, good employee, and good provider. In reality, he felt like an empty shell of a person, literally running on empty.

Little did he know it was about to get worse, He was fired from a six figure a year job. His wife asked him if he wanted to tell his son they were getting divorced or should she? The savings ran out, no income, no love, no spirit, and no hope. When you're 55, your world has crashed, the dreams and hopes gone, and life seems to have left you too far behind, a lot of negative things go through your mind. You begin asking, is this all there is to life. In his final hour of desperation, he heard a still voice say, "I'm not done with you yet. Focus on your heart, on me."

From that moment on, he knew traditional religion would never comfort him. He knew beyond a shadow of a doubt, that if it was going to be, it was up to him. He began searching, learning, asking questions, seeking answers, knocking on any door that his heart told him to listen to. He discovered through trial and error that God did not have an answer for him. He was not punishing him. He was punishing himself.

The search lasted through numerous versions of the Bible, which he considers basic instructions before leaving this earth. He read self-help authors, including Claude Bristol, Eric Butterworth, Jack Canfield, Wayne Dyer, Ernest Holmes, Amit Fox, Billy Graham, Robert Holden, Connie Hopkins, Oakman Dino, Joe Murphy, Joel Goldstein, Norman Vincent Peale, Tony Robbins, Robert Schuller, Wallace Wattles, Zig Ziglar, and others.

Each of these offered stories and advice that sounded very familiar. Further research revealed that each lesson taught by these authors was, in one form or another, found in scriptures—in Matthew, Mark, Luke, John, Psalms, Proverbs, James, and Hebrews.

Something Emmet Fox said kept coming back to him. He stated that to really understand, one must look below the surface meanings of Biblical writings. It was not until he looked below the surface that he found the answers to health, wealth, success, happiness, peace, joy, abundance, prosperity, grace, and gratitude that sets all people free. The Bible's answer: "Be transformed by the renewing of your mind," Romans 12:12.

The question then became: how do I do that? Answer: meditation on getting right inside before I get right outside. Meditation goes deep within and communicates with, believes in, connects with, and sustains his daily life with the infinite intelligence of the universe that he calls God.

Now, in 2009, he's out of debt, except for his mortgage, has repaired and restored his relationships, has created a business from scratch serving others that is prospering, has gained control of medical conditions, and leads a simpler life full of health, wealth, success and happiness, peace, joy, love, grace, and gratitude for all blessings by willing, through his life to bless himself and others. I know this is true, he now sells insurance products; his office is Starbucks; I'm sure he's read over 200 motivational books. I'm learning a great deal from him and he uses spirituality and wellness in combination with his insurance products. He really is a doctor of wellness and insurance for his clients. He's helping people financially and spiritually. Whoever met a businessman like that? I did.

How can one better, his/her life condition and leave a legacy contribution to show others how to reach the highest potential? People who are in the midlife years need help traversing from where they are to where they want to be. Because of all the reading Jack has done and recommendations he has followed himself, he has developed a nine-step after transformation—a meditation to rekindle one's faith, belief, purpose, passions, goals, plans, actions, persistence and gratitude. The idea is to synthesize the thought to re-create, from one's life to leave the world a better place for once having been alive. I include his nine-step transformation, as he gave me permission to do so.

- Belief in a higher power
- Belief in self
- Forgiveness
- Purpose
- Goals
- Plans
- Actions
- Persistence
- Gratitude

Some would say crisis is the mother of the creative process. When you are in trouble, your creative mind goes to work. The creative and inventive mind perks up amid chaos.

Our health is going to hell and we are starting to look to the heavens and the bottom of the barrel.

Lance Armstrong had not won one Tour de France till he developed brain cancer. Now he's won seven, what an achievement.

Breakdowns lead to breakthroughs. Psychological suffering, anxiety and collapse lead to new emotional, intellectual and spiritual strengths that perk the creative mind.

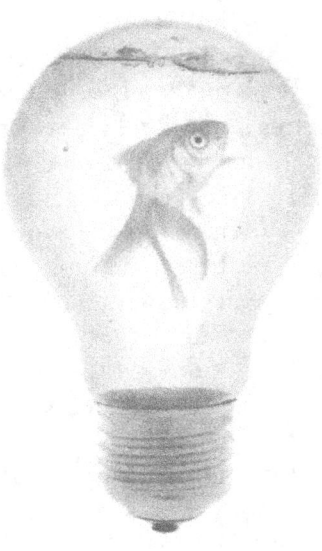

Thomas Edison, the inventor, had 1000 failures before he created his greatest inventions. If what you tried did not make you well, then create another vision and try till you get the job done. Many systems of breakdown are actually harbingers of breakthroughs.

The mother of creativity is dreaming, vision, and chaos. Confusion and death can lead to new scientific discoveries. Don't be afraid of a new idea, or that you are traveling alone, or that no one agrees with you. That's how the creative mind works many times. Announce, "I will be healthy again. I'm not going to die." Write it down and tell a friend. Your affirmations probably will come true.

Sometimes in your life all your attempts at wellness lead to a tipping point, just like Malcolm Gladwell describes in his famous books. Suddenly, all of your attempts at wellness, proper eating, exercise, stress reduction, commitment to develop a purpose and improve yourself-esteem fall into place. You look in the mirror and see that you are there. You created a new person in health. After all that work suddenly, it is there, "your tipping point".

Many believe that psychic phenomena are inventive, a fact, that may bridge the gap between creative genius and clinical insanity. Creativity can result in a lifetime of motivation.

Charles Darwin, the father of evolution, was ill during his trips on the ship, the Beagle. Yet he survived because of his creative genius and purpose to keep them alive so he could write *Origin of the Species*, the genius of his life. Had it not been for his illness, his theory of evolution might not have become his all-consuming passion that produced his great work, a creation from a mind based on scientific studies.

When things are too easy, greatness many times is out of touch. Poor health can be motivating to wellness, survival, and creativity.

I have known many ill and severely injured patients over my 40 years in neurosurgery; a significant number of them have been creative and very successful. A number have been creative to health. Dr. Liz Taylor Witt lost her speech and was paralyzed on the right side following a stroke. She in essence, created herself back to complete health, and then wrote a famous book, A Stroke of Insight.

Look at the Israeli army, 750,000 soldiers defeated 40 million Arabs. They asked their leader, Golda Meir the reason why she knew they could do it. Repeatedly, she said, "No choice." So it is with many of us with serious medical problems in the present or the future. When we have little choice, we finally get down to business and become creative and get ourselves back to health.

One of my patients, who was paralyzed in his arms and legs, invented the Post-it notes and sold them to 3M. He also owned a lot of printing companies.

Hemingway did not write his famous novel till he went through a horrifying war. It stimulated his creative mind. He then wrote *The Old Man and the Sea*. The bottom can be the catalyst to creativity at the top.

Transformation and creativity can occur due to some chaotic situation that shocks us into change. It is when some force deep within us takes over and we will never be the same again.

Catherine the Great, the Queen of Russia, had to be creative, seizing the army to defeat her husband, who was in the process of killing her. She became creative and won the day. People who are threatened with extinction, use the plasticity and spirit of the mind to make a radical transformation and become creative.

When you're growing up in a very unhealthy family, smoking, drinking, obesity, you will need to become educated and creative and visualize a different world for yourself. Why not live the rest of your life in good health, be creative, motivated to change. Don't look back, live in the present moment and visualize a good future.

Look for the "divine fire" in your life, your "creative genius." We all have it. It may be hidden, so look for it! Maybe like Malcolm Gladwell says in his book, *Tipping Point*, it suddenly appears.

What does creativity mean? Creativity involves the perception of new relationships, ways of motivating yourself to health, ways of observing good health, ways of practicing good health. Creativity is not limited to any one domain; it's not just for the arts or sciences. A second component of creativity is utility. It has to be useful and involve some work. Creativity requires action. There is no creativity without action.

They are essentially two types of creative activities. One that is based on our own experience, our own way of thinking, our past history, our own mental processes. It is born out of a logical sequential thought process. There is another type of creativity born out of chaos, the genius type, the new song, the groundbreaking invention, a product of inventors and geniuses.

Neil Simon, the songwriter, was asked how his creative process worked. He said he slipped into a state apart from reality, a dissociative state. "I lost touch with reality," "lost in thought," "intense focus," "another place"—this is a hallmark of the creative process.

He also said, "I don't write consciously. The muse is sitting on my shoulder telling me what to write." Use your imagination when making a plan to wellness. Maybe your real inventive genius will come out; it will suddenly be there. Don't miss the ride. Some creative processes may not be rational or logical. Neil Simon would say, "My mind wanders when I'm talking." I have the same problem. Creative people are usually full of ideas, and many are useless. It's recognizing the good ones that is important. Neil Simon would also say, "Many times I felt like it was invisible." Creative people are all observers of humankind.

We experience own creativity based on our reading, experience, but the real creativity may suddenly appear. Don't deny it, especially if it's attached to wellness.

They have studied creativity with CAT scans of the brain, and it appears to come from many parts of the brain, not just one little center. The creative process begins out of chaos, from different parts of the brain, making links with the present moment, the past and the future. Out of chaos to self organization. Extraordinary creativity is probably different than ordinary creativity. Creativity is not the same as intelligence. One can be more creative and less intelligent and vice versa. Creativity needs action. "Action is my domain," said Mahatma Gandhi, the former leader of India. He said creativity without action is not creativity. One must care about one's health. We are the architects of our own brain. Good health habits are critical. These require, certainly, a degree of motivation. Be creative in your thoughts.

A good night's rest with sound sleep prepares our brain for the next day and renews our mental balance. If repairs our neurotransmitters for the next day's work. It reduces our anxieties, relieves depression and heals our immune system. It motivates us to get out of bed and tackle the

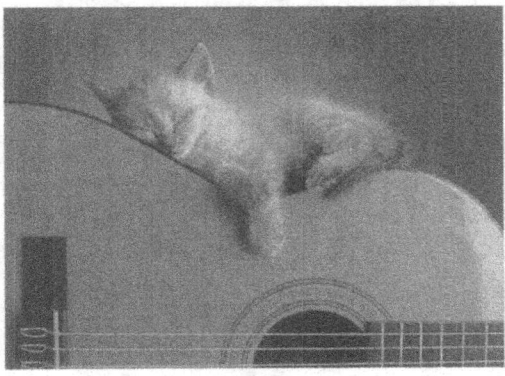

day. After a good night's sleep, you rise feeling refreshed and renewed. Your senses soak up simple pleasures, such as the clean smell of the air, the singing of the birds, and look forward to a cup of tea or coffee. A new beginning, we are reborn after a full night's rest. We look at problems differently, our creative mind works better. Problems that seem insolvable also give us some hope. You are interested in and pleasantly aware of your surroundings, but not overwhelmed. It may build confidence to approach the day ahead, frustrations seem minor, and challenges seem exciting rather than foreboding. You feel more motivated toward the path of wellness, to work out. You are more resistant to eating bad food and willing to start with a healthy breakfast. You can focus your mind like a laser beam on any problem, tackling it with exhilaration and confidence, and you can concentrate at the highest level if your body has had a good rest. If you remember these feelings, you may realize it's been a very long time since you've had them.

We have to be very careful not to accumulate a sleep debt. If you're not getting proper sleep, the sleep debt will accumulate and you will be less motivated. Working out or thinking about what is waiting is much less likely to take place if we are and this sleep-debt mode. There is a great lack of awareness about sleep deprivation. Frankly, it's a national emergency. Not only are we less motivated if we don't get proper sleep, it's also very dangerous, especially when we are driving. We are less creative and less motivated on the job if we don't have a proper amount of sleep. We are much more likely to become ill because of insomnia's effect on the immune system.

When we have sleep debt. We are mortgaging our mind. Incidentally, drowsiness, that feeling when the eyelids are trying to close and we cannot seem to keep them open, is the last step before falling asleep, not the first. It will arrive instantly. Drowsiness is a red alert. Many people have daytime sleepiness, and it can be very de-motivating for learning and work. Also, we are much less likely to go to the gym to work out over the lunch hour, or eat the right food for lunch or dinner. We stop thinking. We want comfort food, the fat, sugar, and salt, the food drugs that feed our serotonin deficiency and make us feel better.

The feeling of being tired and needing sleep is a basic drive of nature, like hunger. If you don't eat enough, you are driven to eat. If you go long enough without food, you can think of nothing else. Once you get it, you eat until you feel full, and then you stop. It is essentially the same way with sleep. Your sleep drive keeps an exact tally of accumulated waking hours. Like bricks in a backpack, accumulating sleep drive is a burden that weighs down on you. Even when you are awake this adds another brick to the backpack. The brain sleep increases until you go to sleep, when the load starts to lighten. In a very real sense, all wakefulness is sleep deprivation. As you wake up, the meter starts ticking how many hours sleep you will need to pay off that night. Generally, people need to sleep one hour for every two hours awake, which means that most need around eight hours sleep a night. Of course, some people need more and some need less, and a few people seem to need a great deal more or less. Each person has his or her own specific daily sleep requirements. The brain tries to hit the mark, and the farther you are from getting the number of hours sleep you need, the harder brain tries to force you to get that sleep.

If you have not met your sleep requirements, it will be very difficult for you to motivate yourself toward proper exercise and eating. There is a big connection between sleep, health, happiness, and motivation.

Your habits will determine your future. Success toward wellness will be determined by good habits.

First let's have a realistic look at ourselves. What are our exercise habits? What are our eating habits? Do we smoke, drink alcohol, use illegal drugs? Do we have a toxic personality? Let's make a list of a good and bad habits. Let's focus on the plan and change things.

What is a habit? It is something you repeatedly do, so it becomes easy. It's your repetitive

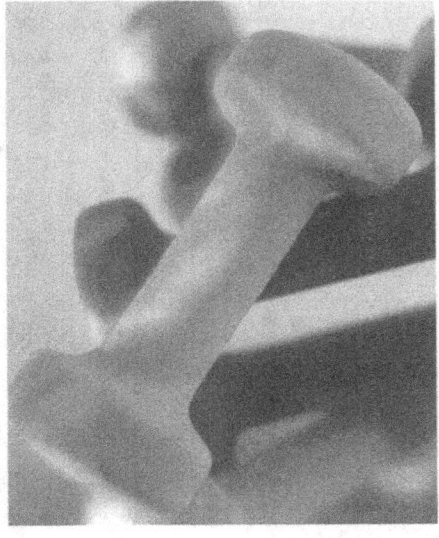

behavior; it's your consistency. If you want to develop a new habit toward wellness, if you do it repeatedly, it becomes automatic. The great news is: you can reprogram yourself anytime. If you choose to do that, it's up to you.

If you're overweight and choose a new way of eating different food, high-nutrient-dense foods, and want to get rid of the fat and sugar habit, it generally takes only about 21 days. If you want to stop smoking, it's about the same period of time.

The key word is consistency. If you repeatedly do the same thing, it will become a habit, good or bad. Don't expect a different outcome if you keep on doing the same thing. Let's call it a no-exception policy. One drink, or one cigarette, or one doughnut and off we go again.

From a health standpoint, if you exercise three times a week to keep in shape, it will soon be a good habit. And you will not be able to live without it. You would do it because you value the benefits. If you want to be in the healthy group of people with good self-esteem and enjoy a healthy long life, your habits will determine your future.

Your habits will determine your quality of life. Riches mean nothing if you're not healthy. I know some people like that, with only a few years to live because of their poor health habits. I know of one that goes to the Pritikin camp for six weeks every year. When he comes home, the rest of the year he again is eating the mad, sad, toxic American diet. Just like anorexics are blinded to the looks of their own bodies, I suspect it is the same for him. Denial will go a long way to destroy your good health. To be rich does not mean just finances, but also good health. You have a lot of money, but if your health is not good, you are not rich. Enjoy your health, your friends, your personal career and family.

The results of bad habits usually don't show up until much later in life. Bad choices can cause a heart attack 10 to 20 years later, but in the majority of people it is 40 years later, including cancer, dementia, strokes, diabetes and heart attacks. A type 2 diabetic has a life expectancy 17 to 27 years less than the average person.

More people than ever are living for immediate gratification. They don't exercise; they watch TV all day, but somebody else running around a sports facility is making himself a millionaire, while they are losing their good health lying on their couches eating fat, salt, and sugar. People with these habits play catch-up most of their lives—from doctor to operating room and a short lifespan. When you develop a bad habit, life will eventually give you consequences. Negatives habits breed negative consequences.

This is a long list when it comes to health that arrives as a result of poor habits. Ninety percent of what we doctors treat is related to our activities, our eating, our stress and how we think. Working 14 hours a day will lead to eventual burnout. When you're eating fast foods or junk foods on the run as a daily habit, the combination of stress and increased cholesterol produces a much greater risk of heart disease and strokes. These are life-threatening consequences, yet many people ignore that and are oblivious and roll merrily along, undaunted by the fact that a major crisis may be looming just around the corner. No wonder 50% of marriages end up in divorce. If you are starving your most important relationship of time and love, how can you expect a happy outcome? You can turn negative consequences into positive rewards if you change your habits. It takes about 21 days to change a habit. About 90% of our normal behavior is based on habits. Once a habit is well developed, it is our new behavior. It can save your life to develop good health habits.

VISUALIZATION

Visualization is the language of the subconscious mind; in essence, it is how we speak to the brain.

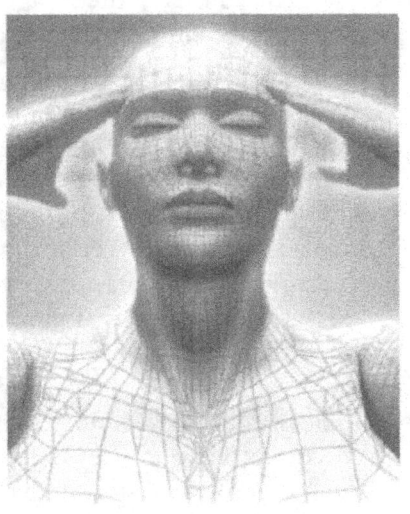

If we create an image of what we would like to achieve, it is more likely to happen. Your brain will not be able to differentiate between what is real and what is not when you speak to it in pictures and images.

It can be very motivating and brings your thoughts into action. The human body contains about 70 trillion cells, and by creating images you are motivating these cells into action.

How does visualization work? Our bodies in the universe are essentially composed of energy. A thought is a quick and mobile force of energy. When we create or accomplish something, we always do it first by using our thought process. Thinking precedes action. Any image creates energy, and having an idea, picture, or thought tends to attract and create that energy form into reality.

We are always attracting the energy of life—whatever we think about the most, believe in the most, or are able to visualize most vividly.

When you visualize your goal, it is much more likely to happen because the act of creating images, or visualization, immobilizes and motivates your 70 trillion plus body cells into action.

Visualization works best after a period of meditation and deep breathing. While sitting in the yoga position or sitting in a chair, take about 10 to 20 deep abdominal breaths and create a picture over your goal. Use all of your senses - smells, feelings, tastes, sounds, and detailed pictures. Do it frequently. If you are visualizing weight loss, picture yourself on the beach during the morning sunrise, wearing great workout clothes, ready to go. Begin your stretch while you smell the ocean air, hear the waves, and feel the warmth of the sun energizing your body. Start your stretching and visualize yourself taking off on a beautiful morning run down the shore. Or imagine that new car, house, or career. You may even imagine doing missionary work and the great feeling it gives you.

When you have the image in your mind, make some affirmative statements to yourself, silently or out loud. "I'm going to lose those 30 pounds; I will have that great job; I will stop smoking; I will stop drinking; I will stop taking so many medications; I will cure my Type 2 Diabetes with proper eating." There are no limits to what you accomplish through the use of imagery and visualization!

The more frequently you do this, and the more detail you give to using your five senses, the most likely you are to achieve your goal. Affirmative statements are very motivating.

Learn to use meditation or deep breathing first so that you are in a relaxed state, this de-stresses your body and you will see the images more clearly. And, you are more likely to achieve your goal as you relax each muscle in your body. Count backwards from 20 – this is a mantra that will lead you into a meditative state. Meditation and visualization will relax you and renew your spirit and can be used during anytime of the day.

Imagery is a powerful and mysterious force in human nature that is able to bring about dramatic improvement in our lives. It is a kind of mental engineering that works best when supported by meditation, and especially strong religious faith. It is not difficult to practice and anyone can do it. It has caught the attention of doctors, psychologists, and "thinkers" everywhere. The word imagine is derived from imagination. Imagery, utilizing the feeling of mental pictures or images, is based on the principle that there is a deep tendency in human nature to become precisely like that which we imagine ourselves to be. An image formed and held tenaciously in the conscious mind passes the present state by use of a mental osmosis and travels into the unconscious mind. Once accepted firmly in the unconscious state, the individual strongly tends to grasp it, and it then becomes part of the individual. The imagery effect on thought and performance is so powerful that a long held vision of an objective or goal could become determinative.

Imaging is positive thinking. Carry this state one step further, and you could say that imaging is a laser beam of the imagination, a shaft of mental energy, in which the desired goal or outcome is pictured so vividly by the conscious mind that the unconscious mind accepts it and is activated by it. This release is so powerful in total force that it can bring about astonishing changes in the life of the person who is doing the imaging.

Let me give you some examples. Jim Thorpe, a famous Olympic athlete, while traveling by boat to Europe never practiced with the athletes on the ship. He never stretched, lifted weights, or jogged. Instead, he sat in the corner, using imagery, about every Olympic event he was to participate in. And, he won almost every track event! He had the used the power of imagery. My race car friend, John Burton, who I play tennis with in Florida once told me a story. Many of the famous racecar drivers imagine the event the night before, using imagery to successfully carry out their goals. Additionally, during the Vietnam War, an imprisoned sergeant, Sergeant Gordon, visualized playing 18 holes of golf every day for seven years. When he was released from prison, during his first game in the United States he shot the best score of his life! That's the power of visualization. I always visualize my serve while playing tennis. And other athletes use this power all the time also. In sports, great athletes visualize what they wish to do, practice the living daylights out of it, and then they don't think when they play the sport, it has now become automatic.

There are four basic steps for effective visualization: to set your goal by tweaking a clear idea or picture, enhance this goal by using the five senses, focus on the goal often, and give yourself positive energy with affirmations of achieving this goal.

For many people, "affirmation's" are most powerful and inspiring when they include references to a spiritual source. There are three elements within you that determine how to successfully create what will work for you in any given situation: desire, belief, and acceptance. These define your intention. Your spiritual source is a supply of infinite love, wisdom, and energy in the universe. Continue to practice your relaxation, visualization and affirmations daily.

Healing

Conscious creative visualization is a process of creating positive thoughts and images to communicate with our bodies - to remove our thoughts out of a place of negativity to a place of positivity, and to replace constrictive and what may be literally sickening thoughts with positive energy.

One can also use visualization and imaging to treat cancer. Dr. Carl Simington published a great book called *Getting Well Again*. In this book, he describes great visualization techniques to destroy cancer cells.

If cancer is your problem this is a great book to read. It has helped a lot of cancer patients. Imaging can also be used to help your pain problems. As a neurosurgeon, I have had a lot of experience with this and it can be very helpful.

The anticipatory power of the imagination has been utilized in many sports, and scientific research has established its effectiveness for athletes. This research shows that by picturing the successful completion of moves they want to make, athletes can improve their performancez—especially if the mental picture is accompanied with physical practice. Good athletes have physical and mental self-control. Jack Nicklaus, author of *Golf My Way*, claimed that hitting a good shot depends 10% on swing mechanics, 40% on set up and stance, and 50% on his mental picture. In his book he describes how to visualize a shot before he makes it; he describes it like making a very colorful movie. He never hit the shot, even in practice, without having a very sharp and focused picture of it in his head. First, he sees the ball, nice and white and sitting up high on the bright green grass. Then the scene quickly changes, and he sees the ball getting to where he wants it—its path, its trajectory and shape, even its behavior on the landing. Just make your movie that shows a perfect shot.

Imagery and healing is probably best known for its direct effects on your own physiology. Through imagery, you can stimulate changes in many bodily functions usually considered inaccessible by a conscious influence. Imagery is a natural language of a major part of our nervous system. It has been shown that the two sides of the human brain think in very different ways. They are simultaneously capable of independent thought. The left and right sides of the brain are different - the right side of the brain speaks in images; the left side of brain speaks more in terms of language and numbers. This essential difference between the two brains is a relatively new way of thinking. The left-brain processes information sequentially, while the right brain processes it simultaneously and specifically.

Imagery in Everyday Life

Imagery has been presented as a powerful device to achieve major goals and objectives. Use it everyday. It can be used to smooth out the minor wrinkles of living. Many famous inventions were produced by the use of imagery. Imagery has its own formula: the goal, purpose, prayer activity, thoughtful planning, innovative thinking, organization, hard work, and always holding the image of success firmly in mind. If this process is faithfully carried out, the desired results will be achieved, despite any and all difficulties or setbacks.

YOU CAN IF YOU THINK YOU CAN

If you have a wellness problem, now or in the future, you come to the realization something needs to be done. Maybe it's obesity, vascular disease with strokes and heart attacks, or type 2 diabetes. Don't feel hopeless or give up, do something about it. Anything is possible. Even if it's advanced cancer, positive thinking and mind-body techniques can double your lifespan and increase spontaneous cure rate—based to my own experience and what I read in the literature. Cancer specialists as a group are just too pessimistic. There are so 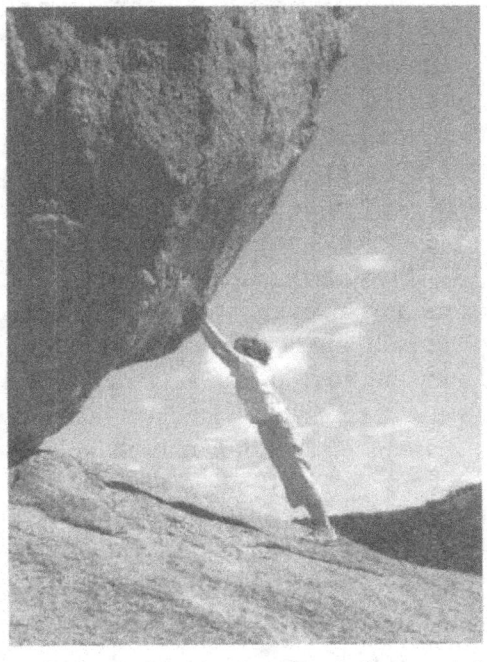 many books on the subject. They fill my library, books on hope and what to do.

When you have a problem, one that is especially difficult and baffling, perhaps unendurable and discouraging, there is one basic principle—never quit. To do so is to admit defeat and your defeatist attitude will come true. Giving up shows a defective personality. It tends to develop a defeatist psychology.

Come at the problem in a different way if the methodology you're using is not working. And if the new approach is not working, come at it another way until you find the key. The computer button that turns on the human brain, your mind, remembers what it is like to be well. Be persistent, it's always too soon to quit.

How do you develop, this undefeatable attitude? You need to develop a program of hope. Throw hopelessness out the window. Don't talk yourself into defeat. It is dangerous to use negative words. No, denotes that you shut the door. It means defeat it delays improvement. Turn things around, and now you have more. Meet the problem.

Change your thinking; meet the problem in a positive, constant optimistic way. Make a plan; write it down. It's motivating.

The refusal to quit is called the persistence principle. Perseverance will win the day—don't be quitters. Send out your positive vision, you cannot create success anywhere in this life without this application of the persistence principle.

Keep thinking positively. Much rain wears down marble. I saw that myself at St. Peter's Cathedral in Rome. If you don't first succeed, then try again. The Perception of all of yourself is critical and is applied by the perseverance principle.

Many times we are our own worst enemy. People can have goals and objectives and work hard and still fail. Perhaps you need to look at yourself and something is amiss in yourself. Sharing what you think may be your personality defects with another person, almost any person, can be of great value. Especially if you bring spirituality into it. Remember attending church is the path to spirituality, no matter what religion.

The hardest person to know is yourself. We have a built-in self-protecting mechanism that always tries to do what we want. It seeks to make the irrational appear rational. Many people will talk about other people and their problems, but they hide from themselves and their own problems.

People who failed usually do that, not because they unable to handle another situation—this is just in conflict with what they've been doing. Remember, if you're doing the same thing again and again, don't expect a different outcome.

You must see yourself as you really are and deal with yourself on that honest basis. That is the perception concept. And it is based on self-examination, a realistic look at yourself because you're nearing the end of the road, or just traveling on the road of poor health and lack of wellness. Stand in front of a mirror and say to yourself, "Now I want the truth about you."

The normal person will realize that self-knowledge is always a beginning of self-development. The process is motivated by perception and releases new powers. It is the road that leads to successful achievement. Plugging away will win the day. Problems are a sign of life. Success weakens you; problem solving strengthens you.

How do you solve a problem, and get motivated to solve the problem? If you acknowledge of the problem, and apply thought and belief, then you have taken a long step down the road to handling it successfully.

Study your health problem; read about it; attend my free lectures; become knowledgeable; then find the weak spot. Break the problem apart, and the rest will be easy. We need the body to carry the brain around. The mind is you. The tendency is to react emotionally rather than to think. The human mind will not think properly when it is hot. Cool it when problems start. Make use of your spiritual power. You can if you think you can, because all the ideas you need to handle every problem are all about you. Cool reactions will open up the lines of communication by which ideas flow to you. The chief duty of a human being is to master life.

To be healthy, vital, and alive, it is very important how you think. To a degree you can think yourself sick, or you could think yourself well. The soul becomes dyed with the color of its thoughts. If you think unhealthy, you will become unhealthy. Think defeat and you will tend to create the circumstances that lead to defeat. You can if you think you can. In the matter of well being, positive results come from visualizing yourself as whole, and you will act on it and get it done.

We may be trying to change something toward wellness, but still don't succeed, because we program ourselves for success or failure every day by the words we say, and the actions we take.

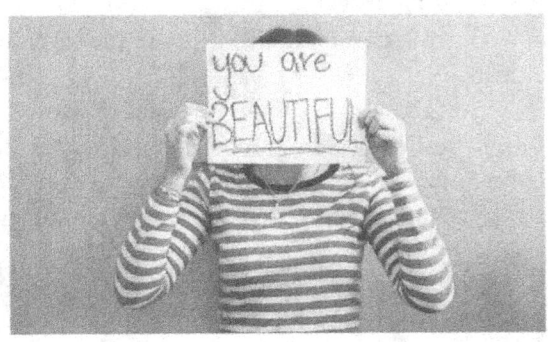

Dr. Shad Helmstetter in, *What to Say When You Talk to Yourself*, says that 70% of what we say to ourselves may be working against us. Seventy-five percent of illnesses are self induced by the words we use. That is exactly my own personal experience in 40 years of neurosurgery. We are everything we choose to be. We are as unlimited as the universe, yet the majority of people fail to achieve their desires and dreams. We sabotage our success by the words we use. Proverbs 23:7 says, "As a man thinks in his heart, so is he." Our thoughts are the words we say to ourselves. Matthew 12:37 says, "By your words, you will be justified, and by your words you will be condemned."

The words we use, whether we say them out loud or in silence, have the power to build up or destroy. We program our success of failure by the words we use. It is your choice. Choose wisely.

Dr. Helmstetter's self-management flowchart explains why our success is conditioned or programmed by our behaviors, feelings, attitudes, beliefs, and verbal programming. This process flows like this:

Programming creates beliefs

Beliefs create attitudes

Attitudes create feelings

Feelings create actions

Actions create results

We are told by self-help authors that we need their motivation. Self-help books are great external motivators. The only type of motivation that lasts is internal motivation caused by the positive words we use.

I teach people to use the statement, "I am." They become what they think.

Jesus used "I am" in describing himself. "I am the Way, the truth, and the light." His purpose statement at John 10:10 says, "I am, that they may have life and have it more abundantly."

It is important that we eliminate all negative words and thoughts from our minds. What we say and what we think determine our destiny. Here is a list of positive statements that I used to offer as help to outpatients to create their own positive self-help "I am" statements:

I am 100% responsible for everything in my life.

I achieve my highest potential.

I live my dreams.

I never settle for less than the best.

I expect the best every day in every way.

I believe in me.

I can because I believe I can.

I can win. I believe I can.

I can do all things through God who strengthens me. (Philippians 4:13)

The universe conspires to do me good.

Everything contains opportunity for me.

If God be for me, who can be against me?

I set and achieve goals that stretch me personally, professionally, and spiritually.

I set goals the night before and focus on doing my very best.

I am health, wealth, success, and happiness.

Everything I desire in my life it is already here for me.

Action is omnipotent. I do it now.

I reject fear and do it anyway.

I do whatever it takes to accomplish my goals.

I ask and receive.

I share with my friends and love their feedback.

I am committed to consistently deliver my best.

Every day in every way I am better and better.

I am positive, loving, and successful.

I finish what I start.

I focus and all the wonderful blessings flowing through me to bless myself and others now.

I embrace change.

I practice truth in all my dealings with others.

I am what I think about most.

I am wonderfully awesome, extraordinary special, and I choose never to be common.

I am worthy.

I am capable.

I am inspired.

I serve others the way they wish to be served.

I focus on my core geniuses.

I say no to that which does not benefit me or allow me to serve.

I have great mentors.

I am a great coach.

I love others.

All the answers I seek are within me.

I listen, learn, and grow.

I always tell the truth.

I am worthy.

I am trustworthy.

I always speak from my heart.

I am thankful for all things.

I am blessed.

I keep my promises.

I am a class act.

I cherish others.

I am frugal in all things.

I give more.

I inspire others to achieve their highest potential.

There are three kinds of people.

People who make things happen

People who watch things happen

People who ask, "What happened?"

The only place where success comes before work is in the dictionary! Let's get to work and become the best that we can be.

It is very difficult to improve your life if you think negatively. It is much easier to motivate yourself if you start your day with a positive attitude. Your brain speaks to your 70 trillion body cells with neuropeptides (300 of them), hormones, and neurotransmitters. Your 70 trillion cells in turns speak to your brain. Mind-body, body-mind. So how you think has a tremendous effect on how you feel and what you might do.

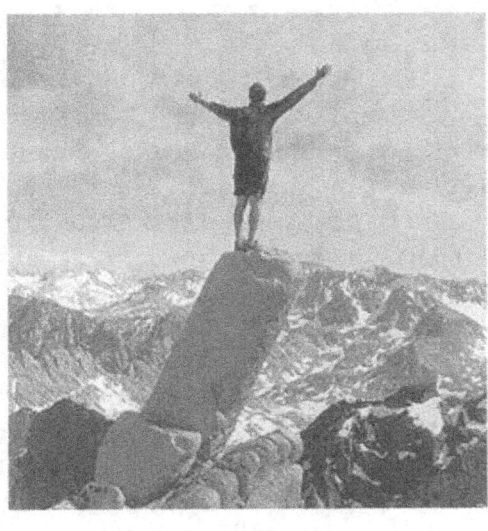

The king of writing about positive thinking is Dr. Norman Vincent Peale. I recommend you read his books. I met one of his assistant ministers a few years ago; he was elderly and said he had all of Dr. Peale books and he said he would never read them again and gave them to me as a present. Many of them were autographed by Dr. Norman Vincent Peale and his lovely wife, Ruth. I am forever grateful. I have read them all, about three times. He would say, "Positive thinkers get positive results." Clearly, he recommends tying your life to spirituality to create life-changing activity. Dr. Peale suggests a number of basic principles that will motivate your life to your goals, and especially wellness.

There is a deep tendency in human nature to become precisely what we imagine or picture ourselves to be. It decides where our life is heading.

Negative thinking is a self-destructive process. He who constantly sends out negative thoughts activates the world negatively. That is the Law of Attraction, which has been widely written about also. Thoughts that are like attract each other. Negative thoughts result in negative results. If your thinking does not change, don't expect a different result. Our thoughts, through neuropeptides, hormones and neurotransmitters affect the immune system and can kill or heal us. Our thought process affects the Intel chips of our body, the eicosanoids, the super hormones. Seventy trillion body cells are greatly affected by our eicosanoids, the communicators. Our white cells make all the neuropeptides our brain makes. Brain-body, body-brain. The positive thinker sends out positive thoughts with images of hope, optimism and creativity.

The greatest discovery of our generation is that human beings can alter their lives by altering their attitudes of the mind. Every problem contains the seeds of its own solution. A positive thinker doesn't react emotionally when in difficulty.

The positive thinker is aware that only by being cool, with strong mental control will produce rational sound solutions. Calm thoughts produce results.

The negative principle negates. You will not motivate wellness. The positive concept will motivate you to change. The positive principle goes for victory. Inspiration and motivation are like nutrition, you have to keep taking daily and in good amount.

Remember there's more strength and power in the individual and his or her ability to change toward wellness. We use only 10% of our abilities on a regular basis our real potential is huge. Write on a card what you intend to be in life; keep the card for constant reference and embed that goal deeply in your mind for a period of years. You will become what you said you would like to achieve.

Motivation is like nutrition. You must take it daily. Remember you're doing only about 10% of what you could do.

Life has an "if" at the center; take control of that. There is magic in believing in yourself. Use imaging and visualization; see your future clearly—what your wellness goals are, what you would like to get rid of in your body, physical and mental fitness—see it. Make a commitment to the principle of wellness. You can if you think you can. Forget the word impossible.

Even if you have only a little faith like a grain of mustard seed, "nothing shall be impossible unto you" (the Bible). Some people are happier being defeated—a sick mental attitude. Don't be paralyzed in your head. Rebuild your motivation; become a specialist in the possible take the "I'm" out of impossible. Remember, faith is the most powerful of all forces. Nothing can get you down if you have faith. Know for sure, there is a giant within you. Then release the giant "YOU".

Don't get down. If you think you failed, just recommit and don't look backwards. The secret of genius is to carry the spirit of the child into old age.

The ability to meet adversity—in failure, sorrow and misfortune—with a smile and renewed enthusiasm for the future is really the secret of life. We're all going to have troubles sometimes. To keep going with enthusiasm at a high level is one of the most exciting things about the positive principle. Failure is only an incident of a successful life. It happens. Get up and develop a new motivational strategy, image and visualize it, and get to work. Keep enthusiasm going in your life now and forever. The words old age or aging are not in my language. "When are you going to retire Doctor?" is a question that really makes me mad. "What are you going to do next Doctor? When is your next book coming out? When are you playing the next tennis tournament?" are better questions.

If you fear inferiority, endure it no longer. Every night free your mind of negative thoughts, like you empty your pockets. Keep positive and nothing will ever be too much for you.

Faith and spirituality are the enemies of fear and are motivating. Form a mental picture or image of the goal you wish to achieve. Dr. Peale would prayerize, visualize, energize, and actualize. This procedure is a powerful force. It's a creativity principle. Goals are dreams with deadlines.

You never know what you can do until you really try—really try. Trying is a continuous process that needs to be sustained at a high level if it is to achieve its goal. Use the power of imagination, creative imaging and visualization, the language of your subconscious mind. Picture your goal and run to it with daily affirmations and positive statements.

Cool it, don't panic. Last year the stock market almost crashed; I was frozen at the computer. I do my own trading. Think hard. Get help. Get motivated. Sitting there panicking, doing nothing, won't do.

The human mind cannot function at its best when it is overheated. Think objectively, not emotionally. Learn to meditate to calm yourself. Get Rudy and Kelly's prescription for stress reduction from our website, *www.kachmannmindbody.com*. Never vaguely and indecisively fool around with a difficulty, take a hold and handle it.

Get in contact with the energy of the universe. The Chinese way of thinking embraces "the Tao", the universal energy, a life-force concept. The truth is we can constantly be in a re-creative process through which the power for life force is ever giving us renewed vitality. Life is energy.

Dr. Peale carried on an extremely active schedule of writing, speaking, editing, public speaking and administration. He kept his own energy and vitality going by constant affirmations of the life force, visualizing it as continuously flowing through his mind. He became tired, but a night's sleep always cured things. Let's face it—he had a highly purposeful life and that is very motivating.

Don't drag through life. A multitude of people drag through life in a dreary sort of way, having little or no zest. They may have very little wrong with them, but life is not very invigorating for them. When a person of this type has a real energizing and vital experience, he is astounded by the new quality of his life. Thomas Edison said, "If we did all the things that we are capable of, we would literally astound ourselves." Empty the mind of all unhealthy thoughts; replace them with creativity. Visualize a life force operating within you, connecting you and refreshing your body, mind and spirit. Affirm it daily with positive statements. Get in harmony with the basic rhythm of life. Connect all your activities to the positive principle. Remember, fear and negativity can destroy; faith and positive thinking can create and develop. Reprogram your thinking and become a practitioner of the positive principle. Then miracles will start to happen. The best is yet to be.

Live your life and forget your age. It's a spiritual experience that really changes things, the in-depth type that brings you to life and keeps your life every day all the way. Develop strong mental shields to ward off the bombardment of negatives. Keep contact with spiritual retreat of power and you will always and forever keep the positive principle going. Think future. I'd like to live to be a hundred years old, and be of sound mind. To achieve that your goal will need to live a life of wellness, physically and mentally.

EXERCISE AND RHYTHM

The concept of rhythm is an integral part of life and is as old as history. Look at the old religions, tribal dancing, Hinduism. Dancing is thought to be the Arjun of the universe. In Hinduism, you've heard of the ancient cosmic dance of SHIVA. In Hinduism, the frequency and randomness of all such sounds are considered to hold healing powers, as is the vocalization "ohm". Apollo, the son of Zeus and the God of medicine, was known as a dancer. In Sparta, authorities require parents to instruct their children in the art of

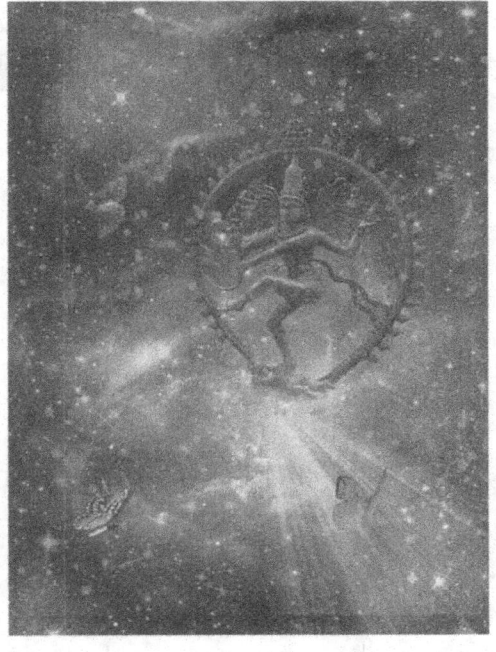

dancing, beginning at the age of five. Dancing is thought to be good for the body and overall health, as well as for the soul. Moving to modern science, researchers have shown that music in rhythm produces measurable healing effects. Music has been proven to reduce stress and anxiety, as evidenced by moldable studies of heart patients who underwent catheterization and other unpleasant procedures. These patients' anxiety levels were significantly reduced when music was played during cardiac catheterization.

The brain uses rhythm to heal. It is important to breathe in rhythm because it affects our immunity. Healers across many different cultures have employed dance to induce a trance as part of a healing ritual. The Chinese discipline known as tai chi, which originated more than eight centuries ago, is still used as a healing art. Tai chi creates a meditative state that is set to restore natural rhythms and balance in the mind and the body. When you combine movement with rhythm, you enjoy the double benefit of exercise and in the meditative state, you lower the inflammatory factors in the blood. It is better when you have a bit of

low-back pain to do some rhythmic movement instead of lying in bed.
What action should you take?

- A 30 minute walk every day, in rhythm
- Swimming
- Entry-level aerobics and advance over time
- Ballroom dancing—I did it for two years with two Russian dancers.
- Biking
- Rowing
- Jogging
- Jumping rope
- Tap, hip-hop, square dancing
- Competitive sports
- Martial arts

Get a personal trainer, when possible.

Learn the dance of life, one of the secrets of motivating yourself to wellness. All types of dance are great. I'm speaking about accommodation of rhythm and movement to improve your longevity and intelligence. You have to use your mind to dance correctly. Ballroom dancing improves the mind and the body. Join a class and do this one or two days a week regularly.

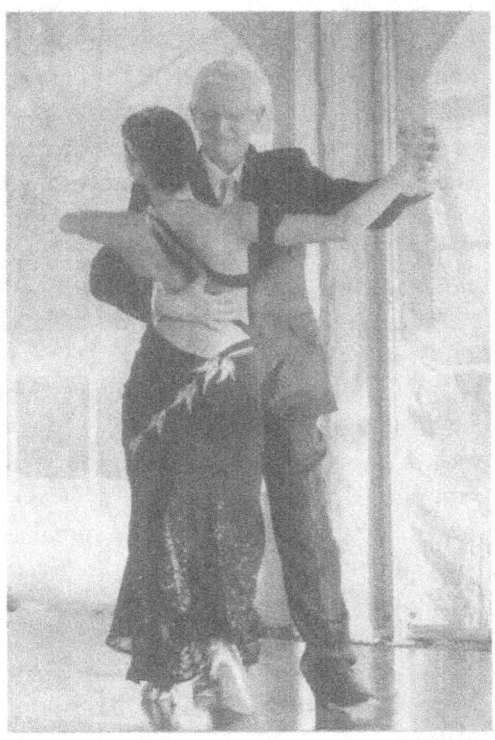

So whenever you are moving in rhythm, whether or not music is playing, you can consider yourself to be dancing. The dances of walking, jogging, biking, swimming, hiking, and even golf or tennis are following a rhythm. Keeping in rhythm means the timing of the swing, shot after shot, so you develop consistency. I play a lot of tennis, have all my life, and really it's a form of dancing.

The effect of exercise on the immune system has been scientifically proven. Scientists have found that exercise has a direct effect on our white blood cells, the main cells affecting our immunity. After a few months of exercise, the levels of immune activating cytokines produced by white cells drop over 50%, while the levels of immune protective cytokines rise about 35%, scientific studies have proven. Exercise is probably the single most effective way to lower inflammatory factors in the blood that cause cancer and vascular disease.

When physical activity is done through rhythm, it can be considered dance, a powerful way to get the most benefit from your exercise program. Pilates for example is an excellent way, as well as all other basic yoga activities. Chi-gong, tai-chi, kundalini yoga, and dancing have the greatest effect on the inflammatory factors in your blood, the CRP (C-Reactive Protein) levels. Researchers have found that the greatest effect on anxiety and depression and benefitted people who performed exercises such as jogging, swimming, cycling, and walking. And music in rehabilitation and physical therapy programs for Parkinson's disease patients also has been shown to improve outcomes, when compared to standard physical exercises. Any rhythm to movement certainly increases the level of enjoyment and involvement in exercise classes. The addition of pumping rhythmic music to aerobic exercise classes encourages participation and increases satisfaction levels. Asked me and I will tell you, I own a yoga studio, and it works for our clients and us. Turning a standard exercise routine into a dance is more fun, less boring, and ensures that exercise is kept at their activity level.

Why does rhythmic exercise works so much better? RHYTHMIC contraction, alternating between flexion and extension, provides balance and strengthens both flexors and extensors equally. The nerve impulses that regulate muscle groups originate from signals in the brain and are transmitted along the spinal cord. With make movement rates of pattern in the brain and spinal cord that is also transmitted to our immune system. The same neurotransmitter chemicals released by a brain and nerve endings are sensed by our immune system. When a brain is dancing, so is our immune system. Human life itself consists of rhythms; it's quite possible that the immune system responds to these rhythms.

SELF-DISCIPLINE AND ENTHUSIASM

Enthusiasm exaggerates the importance of things, and overlooks the deficiencies. Self-discipline motivates you into a realistic direction. Enthusiasm can be wasted energy, and it may not be good. Then again, it does have some value.

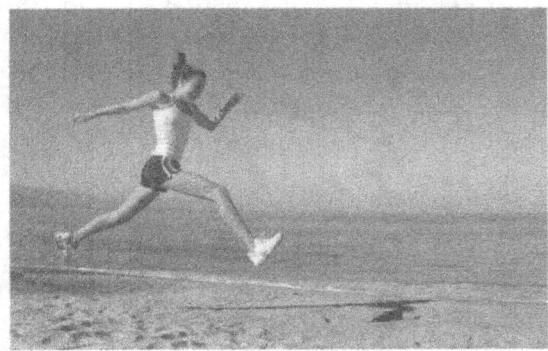

Self-discipline is taking control of your thoughts, habits and emotions. Self-discipline must be done daily. You never master it completely, but it becomes easier with practice. You watch what you eat daily, thought-fully, and eventually it will be a habit and you won't have to think about it every time you take a bite. The same with exercise then, daily, or multiple times per week. After about six weeks it is just a habit, thoughtless and is something you just do, like being nice to people on a regular basis. Complete dedication is the extreme of self-discipline; highly successful people exhibit this trait. If you want a huge change in your health habits, you must have self-discipline and dedicate yourself to get the job done. Small changes are motivating. We all can do that; it does not take a special person. You just have to make up your mind to do it. You must motivate yourself to make the sacrifices. What you eat will walk and talk with you tomorrow. Just think, you could get rid of type 2 diabetes in 30 to 60 days. What a triumph.

Sometimes you need to have self-discipline, dedication, sacrifice, a coordinated plan and maybe a few sleepless nights to turn a bad habit around. The price needs to be paid. You can if you think you can.

The common denominator of success to wellness over another person who doesn't achieve it lies in the fact that you have good habits to do it and the failing person doesn't. The failing person will get obese, diabetes, heart attacks and strokes at a younger age, as well as increased rate of cancer. So the path to wellness is important.

Any resolution or decision you make has no value and is worth nothing until you make a habit of wellness and stick to it. You have to make the change every day, keep it every day, or if you miss one day, you have to go back and start all over.

The kind of determination and commitment required is a good dose of self-discipline and persistence. Anyone can do it if they want to.

The ultimate competition exists within ourselves. What you do will eventually be your habits, and your habits will be your character. Enthusiasm can be overdone. It's self-discipline that gets the job done and is very motivating.

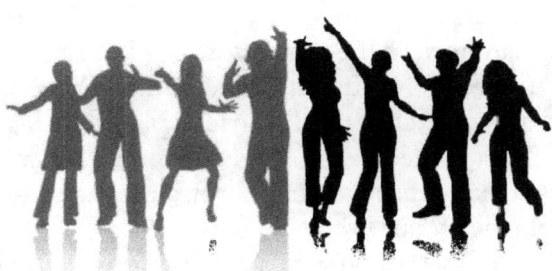

Sound and music have motivational and healing powers leading to wellness. When I turn on the radio in the car, I hear the melodious sounds; I visualize the instruments being played; occasionally I even conduct the music. The stresses of the day disappear. I don't need to stop at a fast food restaurant to get my serotonin up. I can go on to my next project like playing tennis, or a meeting, or working out, and feel motivated. This is much better motivation than food or a pill.

Studies have shown that listening to Mozart increases brain activity and ability to learn. It seems to connect sleepy neurons and awakens neurotransmitters. Music, and especially the music of Mozart, accentuates the learning process For some people it connects the mind and body to wellness. Have you ever noticed the number of people exercising with a Walkman in their ear? The number of people running down the beach while listening to music—they are in heaven. Have you noticed they play a lot of music at the retail stores? They clearly are doing this to increase your optimism and to loosen up your purse strings.

We play music in the hospital to motivate the immune system to promote healing. It keeps the brain balanced and in harmony. The healing power of music brings you into harmony and balance and leads to wellness. The real genius of musical healing lies in teaching the body, mind, and heart to discover and play their own music.

Patients who are dying have been asked why they are singing. They say: as long as I am singing, I am motivating toward wellness, for this is done through neurotransmitters, neuropeptides, and hormones.

Norman Cousins in his famous book, Anatomy of an Illness, describes his visit to Pablo Casals, the famous musician, in his home in Puerto Rico at the time of Casals' 90th birthday. The renowned cellist suffered from rheumatoid arthritis, emphysema and other ailments, including swollen hands and clenched fingers. But as a student Casals labored to see himself at the piano, Cousins witnessed an outstanding transformation.

"I was not prepared for the miracle that was about to happen. The fingers slowly unlocked and reached toward the keys like the buds of a plant toward the sunlight. His back straightened. He seemed to breathe more freely. His fingers settled on the keys. Then came the opening bars of Bach's "music clavier", played with great sensitivity and control. That is the healing power of music, the motivational power of music, working through our neurotransmitters, hormones, and neuropeptides made by our brain and body.

Casals' fingers had raced across the keyboard with dazzling speed, his entire body seemed fused with the music. His shrunken hands became supple and graceful, and completely freed of its arthritic coils. Casals went to breakfast, standing erect, without any trace of the infirmities he had displayed a short time before. For many like Casals, music is a teacher transcending the pains of the moment.

Music sets up a certain vibratory sensation, which unequivocally resolves in a physical reaction that motivates us to wellness and healing.

Music affects the heartbeat, pulse rate, and blood pressure, and usually has effects on our respirations. Using it motivates us to exercise. Dance and yoga with music are very motivating, great activities toward wellness. Music increases our dopamine, serotonin, and endorphins. Music motivates our immunity and increases our productivity. Many different types of music and sound affect us all differently. One style is not for everyone. Sound was our original healing instrument in history. Taking music lessons, dancing, drumming are all motivational activities to a healthy mind and body.

Oliver Sacks said, "The power of music is to integrate and cure—it is quite fundamental." He studied many very neurologically disabled people, but found that number could almost return to normal as long as the music was playing, and sometimes it lasted a few days. A number of neurologically disabled patients still had their musical abilities. As long as music was playing, the Parkinson patients were a lot less rigid, and could walk much better. Playing music will improve your memory. Oliver Sacks would say memory is always there, but it cannot always be retrieved. Music is one method. "Music holds the key to access the system of memory retrieval. It seems to unlock the hippocampus. Music contributes to the recovery of neural functioning in many ways. Neural plasticity, the ability of the brain to learn new things, even in old age, can be stimulated by music and sound. I play music in the operating room and that motivates everyone in the room. Sometimes I've had people in the room ask if we were really at work. The operation went much smoother, was less stressful, and everyone was motivated to work harder.

Bring music into your life; it will motivate you to exercise. Take up a musical instrument, which will motivate your memory circuits and lead you to wellness.

Self-esteem is a fundamental human need. Without it, it is difficult to motivate ourselves. It works its way within us, with or without our knowledge. Self-esteem, fully realized, is the experience that we are appropriate to life and to the requirements of life. Self-esteem is confidence in our ability to think, confidence in our ability to cope with the basic challenges of life. Confidence in our right to be successful and happy, the

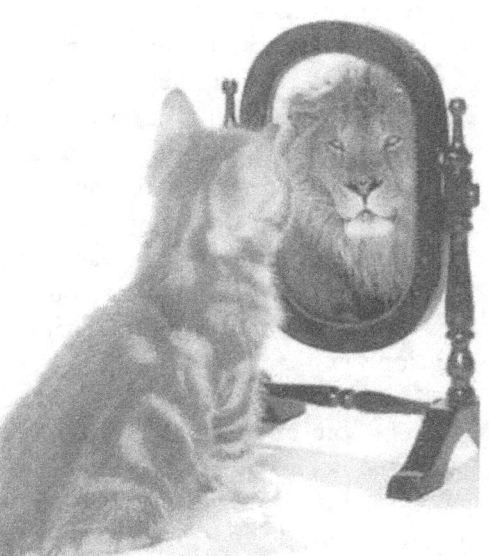

feeling of being worthy, deserving, entitled to assert our needs and wants, achieve our values, and enjoy the fruits of our efforts. Self-esteem represents an achievement, a reward for work activities.

The power of his conviction about oneself lies in the fact that one is more than a judgment or a feeling. It is a motivator. It inspires behavior. It is directly affected by how we act. There is a continuous feedback loop between our actions in the world and our self-esteem. The level of our self-esteem influences how we act, and how we act influences the level of our self-esteem. To trust one's mind and to know that one is worthy of happiness is the essence of self-esteem. If I trust my mind in judgment, I am more likely to operate as a thinking being. By exercising my ability to think and bringing appropriate awareness to my activities, my life works better. This reinforces trust in my mind. If I trust my mind, I am more likely to be mentally positive and bring more awareness to my activities and more persistence to solve the problems in the face of difficulties. When my actions lead to disappointing or painful results, I feel justified in distrusting my mind—the opposite of self-esteem. With high self-esteem, I am more likely to be justified in trusting my mind in the face of difficulties. With low self-esteem, I am more likely to give up, go through the motions of trying without really giving it my best. High self-esteem subjects were more persistent. People. if I persevere, the likelihood is that I will succeed more often than I will fail.

If I respect myself and require that others deal with me respectfully, I send out signals and behave in ways that increase the likelihood that others will respond appropriately. If I lack self-respect and consequently accept discourtesy, abuse, or exploitation from others as natural, I unconsciously transmit this, and somebody will treat me at my self-estimate. When this happens and I submit to it, my self-respect deteriorates still more. The value of self-esteem lies in the fact that it not only allows us to feel better, but it allows us to live better, to respond to challenges and opportunities more resourcefully and more appropriately.

The level of our self-esteem has profound consequences for every aspect of our existence: how we operate in the workplace, how we deal with people, how we are likely to rise in the company, what we plan to achieve, how we fought a love, how we interact with our spouse, children, and friends, our level of personal happiness. Healthy self-esteem correlates with rationality, realism, creativity, independence, flexibility, ability to manage change, willingness to admit mistakes, benevolence, and cooperativeness. Poor self-esteem correlates with irrationality, blindness to reality, rigidity, fear of the new and unfamiliar, inappropriate conformity or inappropriate rebelliousness, defensiveness, overly compliant or controlling behavior, and fear of or hostility toward others.

High self-esteem seeks to channel and stimulate worthwhile and demanding goals. A rich set of goals nurtures good self-esteem. Low self-esteem seeks the safety of the familiar and undemanding. Confining oneself to the familiar and undemanding serves to weaken self-esteem.

The more solid our self-esteem, the better equipped we are to cope with troubles that arise in our personal lives or in our careers, the quicker we are to pick ourselves up after a fall, the more energy we have to begin anew. Most successful people have had a number of failures, but they pick themselves up and begin anew with enthusiasm. The higher our self-esteem, the more ambitious we tend to be, not necessarily in a career, but in terms of what we hope to experience of life, emotionally, intellectually, creatively, and spirituality. The lower our self-esteem, the less we aspire to and the less we are likely to achieve. Either path tends to be self-reinforcing and self-perpetuating.

The higher our self-esteem, the stronger the drive to express ourselves, reflecting the spirituality within us. The higher our self-esteem, the more open, honest and appropriate communications are likely to be, because we believe our thoughts have value and therefore we welcome all the interior clarity. The lower our self-esteem, the more evasive and inappropriate communications are likely to be, because of uncertainty about own thoughts and feelings and/or anxiety about the listless response. The higher our self-esteem, the more disposed we are to form nourishing rather than toxic relationships. We tend to feel most comfortable, most at home with persons whose self-esteem level resembles our own.

What is required for many of us is the courage to tolerate happiness without self-sabotage. Pre-judging is sign of poor self-esteem, and the need to perceive some other group as inferior. Self-esteem, high or low, tends to be a generator of self-fulfilling prophecies. We function better with self-esteem and it is a basic need in all of us. It is essential contribution to the life process. It is indispensable to normal and healthy development; it has survival value. An excess of troubles can surely knock down high self-esteem people, but they're quicker to pick themselves up again.

Good self-esteem increases the likelihood that we will find a way to meet our everyday needs. Good self-esteem has economic value. If we lack adequate self-esteem, the amount of choice offered to us today can be frightening.

Self-esteem has two interrelated components. One is a sense of basic confidence in the face of life's challenges, self-efficacy. The other is a sense of being worthy of happiness, self-respect. Self-efficacy needs confidence in the functioning of my mind, in my ability to think, understand, learn, choose, and make decisions, confidence in my ability to understand the facts of reality that fall within my interests and needs, self trust, and self-reliance. Self-respect means assurance of my value, and the furtive attitude toward my right to live and be happy, comfort in and properly asserting thoughts, wants, and needs, the feeling that joy and fulfillment are my natural birthright. Self-esteem is the disposition to experience oneself as confident to cope with the basic challenges of life and be worthy of happiness.

Self-esteem is a basic need. Our need for self-esteem is the result of two basic facts, both intrinsic to our species. The first is that we depend on it for survival in our successful mastery of the environment and the appropriate use of our consciousness, life and well being, and ability to think. The second is that the right use of our consciousness is not automatic, is not wired in by nature. In the regulating of its activity, there is a crucial element of choice, therefore of personal responsibility. We depend for our survival and well being on the guidance of our distinctive form of consciousness, the form uniquely human, our conceptual faculty, the faculty of abstraction, generalization and integration. In other words, how we think is everything; we are dependent on our mind. The right use of our consciousness is not automatic; it is not wired by nature.

Human essence it is our ability to reason, which means to grasp relationships. It is on this ability, ultimately, that all life depends. How mine includes the totality of mental life, including the subconscious, the intuitive, the symbolic comment, all of which is associated with the right brain. The Mind is all that by means of which we reach out to and apprehend the world. We are the one species that can formulate a vision of what values are worth pursuing, and then pursue the opposite. If we have good self-esteem, we are more likely to make good choices. Look at the choices we have, focusing versus non-focusing, thinking versus non-thinking, awareness versus unawareness, respect for our reality versus avoidance of reality, respect of facts versus indifference to facts, respect for truth versus rejection of truth, honesty versus dishonesty.

The term self-efficacy is a basic power or confidence that we associate with healthy self-esteem, and self-respect to the experience of dignity and personal worth. To be efficacious is to be capable of producing a desired result. Confidence in a basic efficacy is confidence and ability to learn what we need to learn, to do what we need to do in order to achieve our goals, insofar as success depends on our own efforts. Self-efficacy is the conviction that we can never make an error if the conviction that way we are able to think, to judge, to know and to correct errors. It is trust in a mental processes and abilities. In a world in which the total human knowledge is doubling about every 10 years, our security rests only on our ability to learn. The root of self-efficacy is a home environment sufficiently sane, rational, and predictable as to allow us to believe understanding is possible, that thinking is not futile. As far as own actions are concerned, the root is the will, efficacy itself, a refusal to surrender to helplessness, and the quest to understand even in the face of difficulties.

Self-respect entails expectation of friendship, love, and happiness as natural, as a result of who we are and what we do. A concern with right and wrong is not merely the product of social conditioning. A concern with morality or ethics arises naturally in the early stages of human development. The concept comes from adults, from whom you hear the words, good, bad, right, wrong. But the need is inherent in our nature. It is tied to the issue of survival. To be right as a person is to be fit for success and happiness; to be wrong is to be threatened by pain. The need for self-respect is basic and inescapable, inherent in our existence and humanity. Pride is the emotional reward for achievement; it is not a vice to be overcome by the value to be attained.

Self-esteem expresses itself in the face, manner, and a way of talking and moving that projects the pleasure one takes in being alive. It expresses itself in the comfort one experiences in giving and receiving compliments, expressions of affection, appreciation and the like. It expresses itself in an attitude of openness to a curiosity about new ideas, new experiences, and new possibilities in life. High self-esteem is intrinsically reality orientated. Good self-esteem, in realism. You have a respect for facts, and recognition of what is and what it is not. You cannot change what you wish to change unless you have a realistic look. Face it with good self-esteem and develop a program to change. Persons with high self-esteem have creativity, are able to manage change, have independence, have some flexibility and a willingness to admit and correct mistakes. Low self-esteem is associated with fear of reality. To change to a Provo wellness requires a realistic look at the present situation. Then you can be motivated to make the appropriate corrections.

Respect is the degree of value one has for someone else. If the other person realizes that, it can have a great amount of value for motivation. By staying on the same level with the persons or individual we are trying to motivate, we are more likely to stimulate them to wellness.

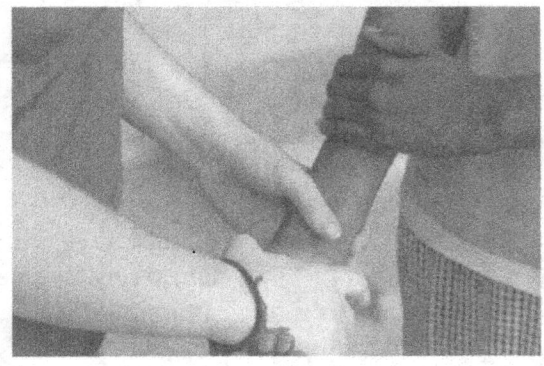

For example, when I'm trying to motivate a group or patient to change what they are eating, their habits, I tell them stories about my own travails and mistakes and triumphs. I bring myself to their level of problems. They know I am not speaking down to them and not pretending to be a perfect person, that I am in good shape, exercise regularly and have normal BMI results. Without respect from the audience toward me, I doubt I would get a lot done.

Also, I'm trying to establish a psychological social relationship with the audience or individuals over time. That increases the chance of them doing what I've asked them to do toward a goal of wellness.

For example, I examined a patient in my office today, trying to get her to change her lifestyle because of a back pain problem that did not require surgery. I don't just see them once and say, "Surgery won't help and you need to lose weight and exercise more," and leave it at that. I see them back before six weeks to see how they are doing, to encourage them if they have lost weight and are doing the exercises, or to reinvigorate them, which is more likely to happen, because we are developing a stronger patient-doctor relationship. They also realize that I really do care about them, and am sincerely trying to help them change to a path of good health—a lifestyle change. I had given my pitch six weeks ago, and I could see she came in today to let me know that she agreed surgery was not the answer. And she was willing to change her ways of eating and exercising. I reviewed the MRI with her, carefully explained that the lumbar degenerative disc disease was from getting a day younger. She laughed and clearly knew what I meant. I always tell my patients that chronic aging diseases are from getting younger. They laugh, and they fully understand what I mean. They leave the office much happier.

When trying to motivate children, it is very important not to hover over them, but instead sit down with them or sit on the floor, and try not to preach to them. They need to know that you respect them and care about what the problem is.

When I'm trying to get a seriously obese patient to change to my way of thinking, I never talk about their cosmetics directly. Their perception or image of themselves may be totally different than what I'm thinking. At most, I might ask them to stay in front of a mirror, have a realistic look, and visualize what they'll look like in six months, after their weight-loss, and to do it often. I usually include a story about my struggles and myself and the patient realizes they are not alone.

Occasionally, I see a prisoner in the office, usually accompanied by a police officer, and am especially careful to be respectful and not criticize anything about them. It was strictly about their health and I tried to complement them about something, and bring myself to their level in some way. I identify with their struggles and look for an opening so that I might be able to motivate them toward health, physically or mentally. It's not because the problems with the law that I'm seeing them, but about problems with their health that I sincerely care about.

When I make the rounds in the hospital, I try to get my body to the level of the patient, not to hover over them. Occasionally I sit on the bed or the floor to get to that level. It's respectful. If a spiritual leader is in the room, I show respect for the individual and asked him to say a prayer with the patient and me, holding hands, for their recovery. It can be very motivating to the patient, because of their own faith, and that I am respectful of their faith. I've done that for many years and find it very helpful toward healing.

I support a group of 60 largely Afro-American and Spanish children from the inner city. We taught these largely disadvantaged children how to sing and dance, and we taught them how to speak Spanish. They are now a very disciplined, motivated group of children. I know we sit in the front row when they perform and their ability brings tears to my eyes. They are well-known in our city. They are the official choir of the Indianapolis Colts. I always bring them up to my patients that live in that area, because it brings me down to the level of the patient. They show me a lot of respect for that, and I am able to heal them much more easily. They realize that I respect them and really care about them, which clearly is the case. Patients show me a lot of respect because they know I love them and care about their state of wellness.

SPIRITUAL MOTIVATION

Sometimes things are so bad that we have to turn to a higher power. That's about what AA does with the 12 step program. But many times we are in a state of non-wellness and not at the bottom. We could still become motivated to lose weight and get in shape by a spiritual connection. With spirituality you would see more love and less fear and anxiety. It would quiet your mind and remove a lot of hopelessness and negativity.

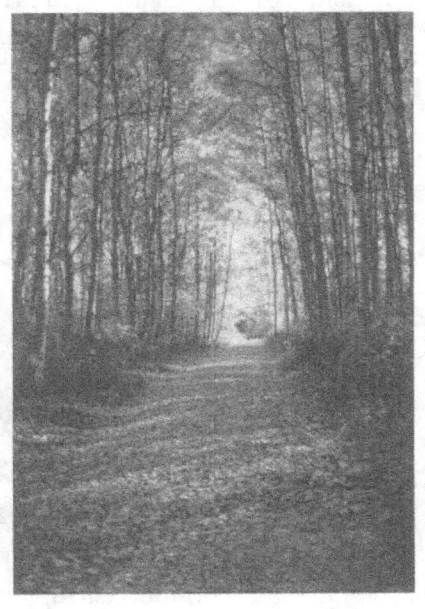

I believe a spiritual connection has great healing power and energy, a path to wellness. Remember, spirituality is the path to religion. It also is the path to wellness.

We have five senses, touch, taste, sight, hearing and smell. But actually, we have six senses and the last one is spirituality. Spirit is the foremost, invisible energy, which is the source and sustenance of life on this planet. This force can be used to solve all our motivational problems to wellness.

When you are trying to take a step in the right direction, you must recognize that a spiritual solution exists and make an affirmative, positive statement in a new wellness direction. "I'm going to lose weight and exercise regularly." "I'm going to get well again." "I'm not going to die from this disease." "I am going to beat this cancer."

In this omni-present, omniscient, omni-potent world there is a solution to everything.

The first step is recognition of the problem: what am I trying to achieve? I'm overweight, out of shape, and have many bad habits, like using drugs, alcohol or smoking. Recognition is the beginning of wellness. Awareness is the beginning of wellness.

Realization is the second step. Create a visualization of the divine guidance you are seeking. Get rid of all doubts. Your visualization will turn into reality within yourself. This is beyond intellectual exercise. With practice and desire in quiet meditation, you will experience the presence of spirituality. You are in connection with the spirit of the universe. Call it God or whatever. It can be a state of meditation, which is pulling you closer to God or spirituality.

Reverence is the third step to a spiritual solution. We know our divinity and commune with that part of ourselves. Faith is healing. In my 40 years of neurosurgery, I have seen it many times. The hormones, neurotransmitters and 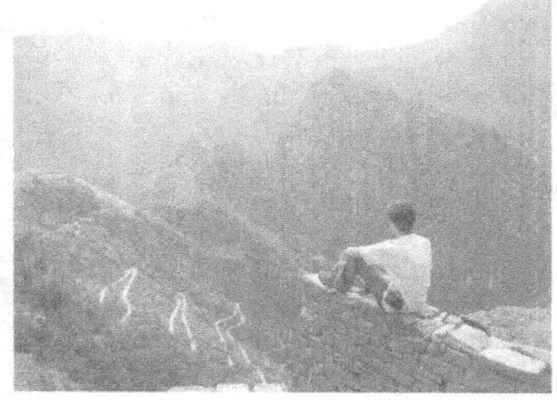 neuropeptides of our brain and body heal us by proper thinking—especially if we believe.

Quietly, communicating a spirituality of God, when we are searching for guidance, is a way of temporarily turning off our ego/mind. Instead of our ego-self thinking I can fix this, we are willing to immerse ourselves into our higher self. Some would say there is a spiritual solution to every problem.

With the divine connection, we are always in touch with a solution. When you practice communicating quietly with the spirit, you will see the Spirit of God. Turn your health problems to a senior partner, God or spirituality.

It is recognizing reality and a reverence that are motivating to a solution.

Dr. Duane Dyer, in his great writings, says the spiritual world is actually part of the physical world. "Spirit is the life of God within us." The physical world is a light bulb, the spirit is the electricity. Spiritual practice is a way of making your life work at a higher level and motivates you to wellness.

Remember, nothing happens, until you make a move in some direction. It's all about your spiritual energy.

The mind with its army of neuropeptides, hormones, and neurotransmitters can heal you. It does it through PNI, psychoneuroimmunology. Thoughts trigger responses by the hypothalamus, (the brain's brain), and the pituitary gland. The 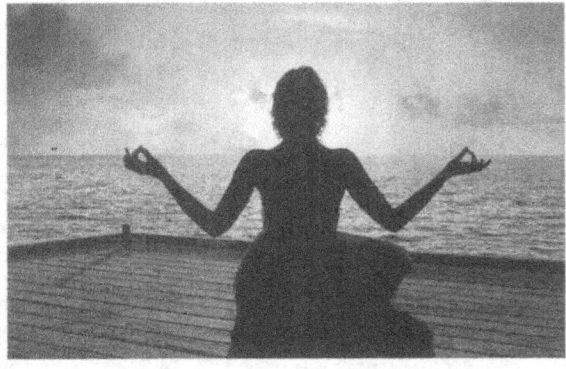 hypothalamus, the Wizard of Oz of your body, can trigger these actions. It's the link between the mind and the body. Positive calming thoughts can heighten immunity, by causing this shifting into healing, rest and repair.

The mind's powerful effect upon healing is so profound that it heals many physical ailments in itself. If your mind is burdened by negative thoughts, you may suffer negative, powerful effects on your health.

I have recommended meditation, breathing, visualization, and exercise techniques to many of my patients. These techniques induce healing and reduce anxiety. I feel certain they are beneficial in many cases. They motivate wellness. I use them myself to lower my blood pressure in the morning. I close my eyes, take 10 to 20 abdominal breaths, say a mantra (mind-body energy), say the words SAT NAM, 10 times. Which brings my mind into focus, the present moment, and I visualize myself sitting at the head of the pier at the lake watching the sun set. Guess what? My blood pressure comes down 20 points every time.

Exercise is the physical element of meditation. That is called kundalini yoga if you do them together. Yoga is meditation. If you pay attention to every body movement you're doing, that is meditation. You can do the dishes as long as you are paying attention and looking at the forks and knives and dishes, concentrating on them, that is meditation. You are in the present moment. You're in the now, nothing before, and nothing after. Your mind quiets down; your brain realigns itself and motivates you to open-mindedness and imagination. Meditation means opening yourself to the truth.

There are many forms of meditation. Transcendental, kundalini, the relaxing reflex of Dr. Benson, the medical meditation of Dr. Khalsa, etc. They are all motivating and will bring changes in your thought process.

Meditation

- Causes calmness—a hypo-metabolic state.
- Reduces blood lactate—a measure of stress.
- Increases serotonin, noradrenaline, and dopamine levels by meditation.
- Decreases indicators of aging, decreased blood pressure, increased vision, increase hearing and improves memory.
- Meditators have 80% less vascular disease, strokes, heart attacks, and 50% less cancer.
- Meditators decrease stress hormones, increase DHEA, increase sex drive and increase the creation of growth hormone.
- Meditators have decreased insomnia—they sleep better.
- Meditators have a 50% decrease in chronic pain.
- Meditation is motivating because you feel better, have increased energy, decreased disease, decrease pain and less anxiety and depression.

What Is Medical Meditation?

Dr. Khalsa designed medical meditation, I highly recommend his book, Meditation as Medicine. He combined kundalini yoga with meditation and called it medical meditation.

It involves:
- Specific breathing patterns
- Special postures and movement
- Mantras specific for each disease
- A unique mental focus

It's very motivating and has worked for many stressed, anxious and painful medical problems. It is ideal for mind-body illnesses.

Dr. Khalsa has assigned specific meditation and exercises for the specific diseases, and then described it in detail in his famous book. The essential mechanism of medical meditation nurtures the ethereal energy system. This is nurturance for the physical body.

Dr. Khalsa, as used for centuries by the Chinese Tao and aurvaida medicine of India, also uses the eight chakras, in medical meditation. They are the energy centers where the lines of energy, the Nadis, lead. Dr. Benson could not separate belief from his medical practice, as traditional medical practice requires Eighty percent of his patients chose prayer as the focus of his meditative relaxation response. Faith is a morning bird that sings in the darkness, anticipating the light of the dawn.

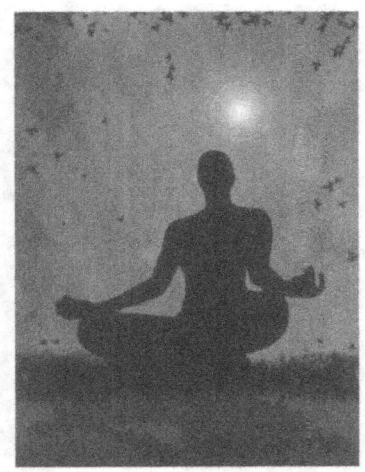

Dr. Benson from Harvard found that meditation causes decreased blood pressure, decreased heart rate, more relaxed breathing and a better mental state. So he called it the" relaxation response." He is known worldwide because of it.

Four Things that Could Elicit the Relaxation Response

- A quiet environment
- A passive attitude
- A comfortable position
- A mental device

The Relaxing Medical Response

- Repetition of a word, sound, phrase, prayer, or muscular activity
- Passively disregarding everyday thoughts that inevitably come to mind and returning to your repetition
- Sit quietly in a council position.
- Close your eyes.
- Slowly and naturally and say some words, sound, phrase, or pray to yourself as you exhale. Continue for 10 to 20 minutes.
- Practice the technique once or twice daily.

Every person has a mind-body connection. So self-care techniques, like medical meditation and the relaxation response of Dr. Benson, can be motivating and have great value in healing.

MOTIVATION AND BREATHING

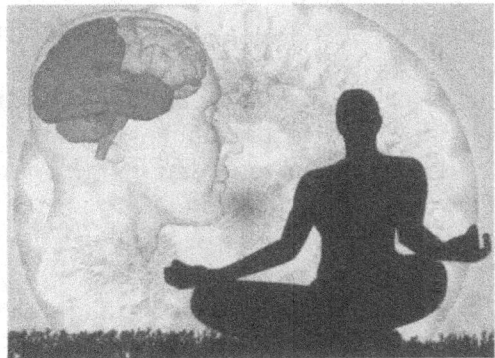

Many breathing techniques lead to wellness. The ancient Chinese, the Tao and the Hindu-yoga traditions, use breathing techniques extensively to achieve a quiet state of mind-mindfulness. That leads to good health and stress reduction.

The Buddha gives simple instructions that form the basis for breath meditation. The meditator assumes the Lotus position, "cross-legged posture". The only time that mindfulness can happen is in the present moment; if you think you know the past that is memory. Mindfulness is unbiased. It is not for or against anything. When you focus on the breath for a few moments, thinking calms itself. Therefore, you could be doing anything, walking, combing your hair, doing the dishes, if you are concentrating on your breath, this will lead to mindfulness. It's meditation.

When we focus on the breath, we are focusing on the life force. Life begins with the first breath and will end after our last. To contemplate breathing is to contemplate life itself. Ancient India had a tremendous respect for the breath, a deep understanding of its powerful effect on the body and mind. In fact, all of the Indian spiritual sciences had some form of pranayama, which is usually translated "breath control." Most forms of pranayama, yogic breathing, involve controlling the breath. The quality of the breathing does improve; it becomes fuller, freer and calmer, with consequences both physical and psychological. We're all breathing. We need to be aware of the simple sensation, the in breath and the out breath. We note that a deep breath relaxes the body and figure that an accomplished meditator will be breathing deeply all the time, period. If we allow the breath to unfold naturally, without tampering with it, in time we may be able to do that with other aspects of our experience, we might learn to let the feelings be, let the mind be. Using meditation in its extreme form allows you to develop a Zen mind. The ultimate goal, the Zen mind is not easy to achieve and takes time to develop.

The breath is an ideal vehicle for teaching Buddhism in the West. It is not religion. It's a way of being. A mindful way of life that leads to wellness.

For some people breathing it isn't a terribly pleasant process. A lifetime of faulty breathing, often accompanied by emotional blockages, has made the breath an unattractive object of attention. You need to develop a certain devotion to your meditation, like counting to 10, or repeating the same word to quiet the mind, in combination with the breathing techniques. Pick a time of day in a quiet place; it could be anywhere. You can meditate sitting at the stop light, or cleaning the toilet.

An excellent way to relax is to concentrate on the breath when taking a walk. It's meditative and leads to healing of the stressful mind. At the beginning and at the end of a walk, stand and breathe mindfully for a few moments. Pay attention to every aspect of breathing, the nose, the lungs, the diaphragm and the abdomen. Breathe like a baby, so the belly hangs out when you breathe in deeply. Pay attention to every part of your body and your surroundings—it's meditation. St. Francis of Assisi said, "It is no use walking anywhere to preach unless our walking is our preaching." There are five rewards for one who practices walking meditation: you can endure traveling by foot, you can endure exertion, you become free from disease, whatever you have eaten and drunk becomes well digested, and the concentration you win while doing walking meditation lasts a long time. It's this concentration, and the joy of walking in such a state that is the primary reward and a state of wellness is close behind.

Sometimes the breath is very fine, like silk or satin; it enters and exits freely. And other times it is coarse, more like burlap, and fights its way in and out. Sometimes the breath is so deep in its root that it affects the whole body, relaxing it profoundly. As you pay attention to breathing, the quality of the breathing changes, perhaps because thinking is diminished. The breath becomes deeper, you find it more enjoyable, and the body starts to reap the fruits of that, to become more relaxed.

It just reflects the power of mindfulness. If your mind becomes angry, all worried, your heart starts to race, your body grows tense. But if you can just be with the breath for while, not suppressing the emotion, agreeing with it, all changes. The mind becomes calm. As the breath goes, so goes the body. The first law of Buddhism is that everything is constantly changing. So your breathing technique can change from time to time. Breathing leaves all the troubles behind, all the preoccupations, worries, plans, doubts, fears, all the stuff that makes up the mind. Especially in the modern world, where everybody is so impressed with variety and complexity, so desperate to be entertained, it is a relief to settle into the simple repetitive act. The opportunity we have of staying with the breathing, consciously coming back to it, is a chance to do one simple, ordinary thing well. Entry into the spirit of repetition can be a powerful lesson in simplicity, which is desperately needed in the modern world. Many people come to meditation expecting some com-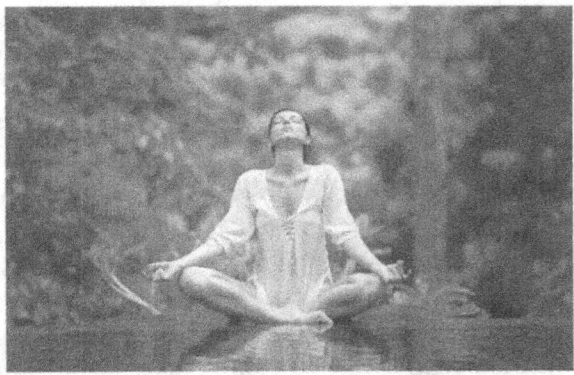plex practice leading to an ordinary exper- ience. They can't believe they're just supposed to sit there and watch the breath. We begin to see how useful the skill is in other aspects of our lives. The constant repetition of going back to the breath has real value. In some ways this entire practice is everything the Buddha said, is concerned with having an infinite respect for life. The practice of breathing and meditation constantly reminds us that everything is worthy of attention. To be mindful of anything is an act of generosity. You are giving it life by allowing it into your world. But the greatest benefit is that you respect for your own life.

The breath is a vital conditioner of the body. The body, mind, and breath become one, and you are able to sit for a long time without pain or discomfort. It's important to emphasize that this process unfolds in different ways for different people, that it generally takes place over a long period of time, that for all, or most, of us it is the fruit of a great deal of sitting. It will cause us, though, to pay much more attention to what we are doing and get rid of destructive behaviors like overeating, lack of exercise, smoking, drinking and using drugs. All of the Buddha's teaching, it has been said, can be reduced to one, under no circumstances attach to anything as me or mine. It isn't that we shouldn't experience rapture or happiness, but that we have to be careful not to attach anything to them.

A huge amount of fear, anxiety, apprehension, is stimulated by thought itself. That is what you are trying to avoid by paying attention to the breath and developing relaxing mindfulness. A usual reaction to fear is to create a battlefield. Our fear is that war, with our tremendous yearning to be free from it, and the state of battle is the mind and the body in which the process is taking place. We tie ourselves into knots, turn ourselves inside out, fighting that battle. The attitude of practice is to open the process up, to see that it's all part of us, the fear, the yearning to be free of it, the mind and the body, the mindfulness observing them, the conscious breathing that nurtures the mindfulness. We sit there with all of that, all one thing. Then one day it comes up; our attention meets it, becomes one with it, allows it to blossom, which is what the fear wanted all along, and then you can get rid of it. It is when we prevent the blossoming of fear by ignoring its presence, that fear hangs around, drags us down, because we spend so much energy holding it off. Even in the blossom, life has its parts. That way, you have all the energy you would have used escaping it to combat it. We also have the energy of the fear itself. It is a great gain in energy when we let things happen. The ground of fearlessness is fear. In order to become fearless, you have to stand in the middle of your fear. We shouldn't trust any fearlessness that doesn't have that as its basis. The beginning of that is to see your fear and admit to it. You acknowledge that you are afraid, and then have the immense courage and humility to study it. It can be the beginning of the end of it. In other words, make a plan to get rid of it. Don't try to suppress it.

Mindfulness and breathing techniques are the road to freedom of the mind.

The process of breathing shows us a way to let go of the old and be open to the new. The process of reading is a living metaphor for understanding how to expand our narrow sense of ourselves and to be present to the healing energies that are both in and around us. Some people say that the diaphragm is the" spiritual muscle". It lies at the foundation of healthy breathing. Shaped like a large dome, the diaphragm functions as both the floor of the chest cavity and the ceiling, all the abdominal cavity. When we inhale, the diaphragm normally contracts. This pump-like motion creates a partial vacuum, which as you know, draws air into the lungs. When we inhale fully, the diaphragm can double or even triple its range of movement and massage the stomach, liver, pancreas, intestines, and kidneys, promoting intestinal movement, blood and lymph flow, and the absorption of nutrients. The work of breathing starts with sensing the inner atmosphere of our organism, the basic emotional stance we take toward ourselves and the world.

Learning how to observe the mechanism involved in breathing, as well as the various physical, emotional and mental forces acting on them, depends in large part on learning how to sense ourselves, to listen to ourselves, to expand our attention to include the sensory impressions constantly arising in our organism. We have to learn to listen to our body.

THE BREATH

In many traditional cultures, the breath is envisioned as a direct manifestation of the Spirit. It is the energy of the Spirit that enlivens us and we received this energy from breathing. The people in India call it the prana, and the exercise pranayama. The Chinese call it life energy—Chi. We are dependent on this life's energy, Chi. Through our breath, we are connected with this life force. Western scientists reject such a life force.

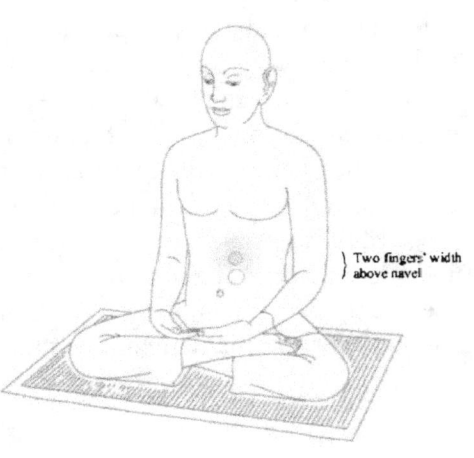

Two fingers' width above navel

It is today, after the documentary success of certain forms, alternative medicine, mind-body medicine, including meditation, and Chinese healing arts such as acupuncture, that a few open-minded pioneers in the West have begun to accept the possibility of chi. It has been popularized by the TV journalist Bill Moyers' PBS program, "Healing of the Mind," which documents the latest breakthroughs. They talk about the mysteriousness of the "chi."

Besides, we are destroying patients with our mortal addictive drugs and medications, and injections and operations. Pain centers in general are "cash cows" that addict people. We need an alternative. Chinese and Indian ways of healing would be an excellent addition to medical care. It could heal 50 to 75% of our people, much cheaper and safer.

Since the birth of Christ, Taoists have been doing remarkable things for the human body and mind through breath, posture, movement, visualization, sound, and meditation. They've discovered how to beneficially influence, not only our thinking and feeling, but also our internal organs, hormones and blood cells, leading to wellness and healing. Many of these practices have been verified scientifically. Research has shown the remarkable influence of Chi on everything from crystals to the human immune system. The Taoist believes we have "three treasures," the "earth form," "cosmic force," and "universal force." These three forces manifest the "three treasures", essence, chi/life force, and spirit. It is the interaction of these forces that determines our life. If the Spirit leads, all three work together very well. If the essence leads, it damages all three.

Our healing and wellbeing depends on the constant harmonious movement of energy, of Chi, throughout the whole organism that Taoists believe comes, not from just food and air, but also from the universe of stars and planets. The Tao regulates the spiritual and physical life as a path to good health and wellness. I believe the Chinese and Indian ways of healing have great benefits, are safer and cheaper. I see complications of Western healing every day, from unnecessary surgery plus too many medications.

FEAR OF DEATH AND ILLNESS

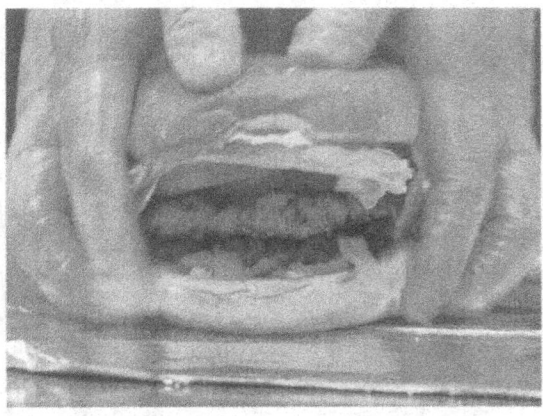

Some of us are only motivated if the gun is pointing at our head. Remember, different things motivate different people. Certainly, in my 40 years of neurosurgery and medicine I have seen a great variety of motivated behavior. One person reacts to a threat in the future and another only if they are facing certain death. You tell one he might get cancer in 10 to 40 years and he won't change, but now he has cancer and that's when he stops smoking, when it probably is too late and he might as well enjoy himself the rest of his remaining days.

When I asked a neighbor at my lake cottage if I could use his huge lot to park cars for my 35th year in neurosurgery celebration party, he told me that he had a very serious medical problem and asked for my advice. He had a failing heart and needed a heart transplant. He said he did not want to go through that, as he was overweight, 60 years old, and he thought God would not let him down. I said, "Max, you got to do something and set a new goal for yourself." I got him the books and DVDs of Dr. Dean Ornish. For many years he has published great books on preventing and reversing heart disease. I've read them all. I'm sorry to say, I have spoken to many cardiologists who know of him but have not read his books. Max followed the recommendations of Dr. Dean Ornish very closely—high nutrient-dense, vegan way of eating, exercise and meditation. Fifteen years later, at age 75, Max builds houses in Marion, Indiana. The threat of death within the year, and the doctor who educated and helped motivate him caused Max to motivate to wellness. He lost about 30 pounds, developed a purpose in life, went back to work. I asked Max how he handled the stress. He said, "Doctor, God takes care of my stress. I have no stress." Very interesting, especially since Dr. Dean Ornish strongly recommends spirituality. Max looked death in the eye and said I will have none of it. Hopelessness turned to hope.

The work of Dr. Dean Ornish clearly explains vascular disease, and the behavioral science behind it and what he recommends. We teach the same way of eating at our wellness studios.

About a year ago I saw a type 2 diabetic with unbearable pain and numbness in his arms. He had diabetic neuropathy. His family doctor called me because he couldn't handle this supposedly belligerent patient. He was unruly because of unbearable pain. When he was better, he had a great personality. Instead of talking about the pain he was having right away, I asked him what was going on in his life. He was retired. He said he played the piano almost every day, but could no longer do it because of the pain in his hands. I told him I was taking piano lessons, and we compared notes. He said he weighed about two hundred forty pounds; his blood sugar was between 200 and 300. I reviewed his way of eating and it wasn't very good, as expected.

I told him we could probably eliminate this type 2 diabetes in 30 days if he followed my way of eating. No calorie counting, no portion control, low glycemic index, complex carbs, whole grain, vegetables, salads, legumes and fruit, all-you-can-eat. Avoiding meat, fatty cheeses and processed food. He followed my recommendations to the hilt. I also recommend daily exercises, and he did that, the 30 minute walk and some mild weight lifting. He came back to see me in 30 days, and it was like a miracle. No arm pains, no hand pains and the numbness was a great deal less. Off medications, and I was looking, frankly, at a very happy guy. I was able to motivate him and he believed me. And he clearly realized that I cared about him. That second visit we spent two thirds of the time talking about piano music. On the first visit I had educated him a lot about what diabetes does to the body, the blindness, the extensive vascular disease, amputations and kidney transplants. I do think that helped motivate him.

So facing illness or death does motivate some people, especially if the doctor does his job. Incidentally, the word physician means teacher. I also had told him he would probably become impotent in a few years if he didn't change his way of eating. That probably was a little motivating, too. To learn that type 2 diabetes is curable 90% of the time in 30 to 90 days, when your BMI returns to normal, certainly also is very motivating to many people. Many of the patients I speak to have never heard of that before. But I stand behind those words. I've seen it and I have many books behind me that state that. The patient also is playing the piano again. That certainly made him a lot happier. As he left the office a second time, he turned to me and said, "Doctor, you are now my coach." I tell you, that was a good day for me.

I've seen a number of substance-abuse patients over the years, as you would expect. They got themselves into major accidents because of mental impairment from alcohol, narcotics, causing death, paralysis, paraplegia, quadriplegia. About 20 to 30% of those that survive generally call it quits on substance-abuse or seek treatment. Injuries can be motivating and changes the behavior of some people.

One husband, though, killed his beautiful blonde wife with secondary smoke. She did not smoke. He smoked in the house and went right on puffing after that. I thought he probably would be living by himself the rest of his life.

Since smoking is still fairly common, I see patients frequently with lung cancer that spread to the brain. Many times, the whole family smokes. Many times after surgery on one of these patients, I have to look for the family outside the hospital because all are standing there smoking. Generally very nice people, but it's a horrible sight, because I can visualize their future. At that point some of them will stop smoking because of what is happening to grandfather, father and now the children. I indeed have been around long enough to see all three die.

Television commercials showing the complications of major diseases do motivate some people to change their behavior. Sometimes a scary TV commercial can do it.

I used to give a lot of lectures to troubled children of high school age. Most of them were stressed out about their personal problems. Ninety-nine percent of them smoked, and their classmates said the other 1% was lying.

I offered a large pizza to any one of them who would stop smoking for one day, none did. A couple girls did so when I told them they'd be looking 20 years older than they really are, as is typical of smokers. The effects on physical beauty can be motivating, from effects on the skin to obesity. It is difficult to convince children to change their behavior, because the future is so far away, especially if the parents have the same bad habits.

There is a group of people that is very difficult to motivate. That is the patients I've seen with Buerger's disease also known as thromboangiitis. They had a very serious vascular disease completely unrelated to nicotine. When things get serious, it starts affecting their toes, their feet, their lower leg and then the upper leg. Stopping smoking would stop the process, but the majority still doesn't do it. And it's difficult to believe or even understand how they can watch their bodies disappear because of that little cigarette. You think you'd almost have to put them on an island with no access to nicotine. I think these patients probably need cognitive counseling or a relative or friend who lives with them who can motivate them daily. It again exemplifies that different things motivate different people, whether it's an illness or death facing them. Even in the face of certain death, some people do not change, unfortunately. Education and a loving family and health care provider certainly can help.

Behavioral Cloning

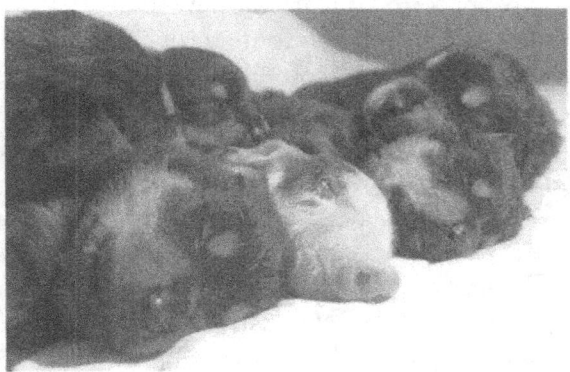

If you can establish rapport with an individual, you are more likely to motivate them. It is the experience of being in agreement with someone you trust. When a person is in rapport with you, he or she is inclined to concur, cooperate, and collaborate with you. If you are trying to motivate them toward wellness, you can see how that would be a lot easier. It will help you create an environment of agreement that might motivate the other person. In essence, we are trying to get the other individual to be a copy of us. It is natural and evolutionary in nature; we copy our own cells and DNA everyday. Behavioral cloning is the reproduction of the language, posture, and pacing of another person. Tamra Lowe, a person who publishes a great deal on motivation, writes about that in her great book, *Get Motivated* and I suggest you buy it and read it. Rapport is a powerful means of establishing trust and understanding with others.

In my own experience, if I can get the patient into a group, they share similar activities and behaviors and are much more likely to do what I recommend. It is in our DNA and genetic structure to respond to group psychology. Our ancestors lived in groups in caves and forests. People who are in rapport usually demonstrate well-matched communication styles and body language. In order to communicate effectively with others, it helps to create a base where people feel understood, appreciated and safe. You are able to bring their habits and activities into alignment with others. But speaking to a child or any person, it is good to get yourself down to their eye level to improve the communication style. I remember when a famous world violinist, Andre Reiu, spoke to my ninety-year-old mother backstage while she was sitting in a wheelchair at a concert. He got on his knees to talk to her. I have a picture of that hanging in my home; that was very motivating to her. She never forgot that moment.

The next time you want to motivate someone to take action, match that body language, tonality and pacing. If they're speaking at a fast pace, pick up your pace when you speak to them. If she is seated at a table with her hands folded, have a seat and do the same. Conforming your posture and communications style to that of the person you are speaking to will help create unity by making the other person feel accepted and understood. Remember, you are matching their style, not mocking them. You don't want to mirror their behavior, just to model it. Your voice, gestures, and body language ought to be similar but not identical, it may motivate respect and may stimulate micro-neurons. Things to watch for: posture, body language, gestures, facial expressions, and eye contact, to show voice, tonality, rhythmic beat, volume, and words in phraseology. When you're trying to motivate and inspire groups, you must appeal to every motivational style. You need to offer something for everyone, so you must know your audience.

Motivating Children

Generally motivating a child is up to the parents, but let's face it, we live in a village. We all bear some responsibility for the future of our society. Whenever I see a child as a patient in my office, as the doctor of that patient I take the opportunity to speak to

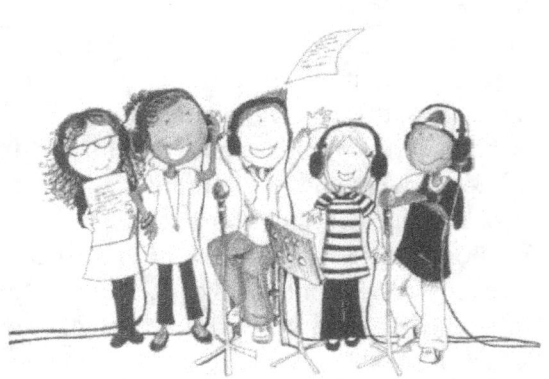

the child. It depends on the age of course. But even a three- or four-year-old can be very interesting to talk to.

The other day I had to speak to a sixty-year-old grandmother's large family about her having a malignant brain tumor. A very serious life-threatening subject and the news was not good. I spent a lot of time with them. Standing in front of me was a four-year-old, a very pretty little girl, and I thought I'd change the subject a bit. Speaking to her, I asked her name and asked, "What are you going to be when you grow up?" Without hesitation, she said. "A mother. And I have already picked out my baby in a magazine." The attitude of the room changed in a second, and there was a lot of laughter.

Whenever I see a teenager in my office, I always asked them what they're going to do with their life. I've given a book of a success story to the teenager a number times. *Gifted Hands* by Ben Carson is a good example. It is a very motivating story of a young black man who was last in his class in Detroit, but his mother, who couldn't read, recommend that he go to the library. He started reading everything he could get his hands on and ended up being a famous neurosurgeon at Johns Hopkins University. A great book to read. When I was a 10-year-old, my German mother handed me a book to read about a famous German surgeon and to this day I can remember him standing there in his white coat. That is the day I decided to become a doctor. So it takes a community, but it's the parents who are mainly in charge.

The best thing we can do is motivate a child for proper diet, plans for the future, put a dream in their minds, and get them to exercise frequently. What the child will do is determined by us and how we deal with them. A good 80% of the time, if we eat a poor diet, what do you think a child will do? Who buys the food in the house? What type of food are they eating at school? It's the mother most of the time. Then again, today mothers are not only raising children, but also working and then the big kid comes home, many times not taking much responsibility for the children himself. In these economic times, it's almost understandable, but unfortunate just the same. Ten-hour days at work, one to two hours trying to get home, and then family responsibilities. We are living in a society where two thirds of adults are overweight; one third of the children are overweight, and many are obese. Most of us are eating the mad, sad toxic American diet.

I suspect if you're lying on the couch at home and watching ballgames all weekend, your child probably is doing no different. Exercise is a very important part of wellness. In adults, it's about 30% of weight loss and maintenance. In children, it's even more important, as much as 30 to 50%. For an overweight child, exercise can be torture. That's why the topic of exercise must be handled with sensitivity and understanding.

The best way to start an exercise program for your child is to look into the child's unique interests, walking, skiing, basketball or tennis, perhaps. I remember an overweight child seeking out one of my tennis friends, who was a high school tennis coach in Peru, Indiana. The boy said his friends were making fun of him and he wanted to learn the sport. My friend asked, "Are you willing to practice two to three hours a day?" The boy answered, "I will." By the time my friend was finished with him, he made it all the way to the Notre Dame tennis team. So a personal choice by a child and a great teacher got the job done.

Not all overweight children who take up sports will become star athletes. As parents, we shouldn't put those types of expectations on a child who is naturally drawn to sports. His or her lack of interest or ability could disappoint, causing a drop in self-esteem. You never know what activity might spark interest in your child, so keep on trying and searching.

The child should exercise 60 minutes a day on a regular basis. It will increase their basic metabolic rate and burn off a lot of excess calories that might cause obesity.

Lack of exercise in your child, some people call child neglect. The overweight child, whose parents are waiting for him or her to slim down as she grows older, is actually a victim of neglect. You're not encouraging your child to grow into a healthy, secure adult. You must motivate your child away from a sedentary lifestyle as early as possible. Playing sport games with your child at an early age is a good way to start. I taught all my children baseball, tennis and swimming, as well as a love of nature. Exercise must be made fun. If you exercise, so will your child. If you watch in ballgames all weekend, so will they. Don't watch television, be your own television. If you want a healthy, secure child, you must find a physical activity that you can enjoy together by either participating with your child or taking a child to the activity and cheering him or her on.

Provide opportunities for safe, active play inside and outside the home. Expose children to as many different kinds of physical activity as possible. Enroll children in sports clubs. Organize activities with the entire family at least once a week. Encourage walking or cycling to and from school. Encourage walking the stairs rather than taking the elevator. I try not to use the elevator at the hospital. Limit time watching television or playing computer games to less than two hours per day. Only allow children to watch television if they have been physically active for at least one hour that day. Don't allow televisions and computer games in children's bedrooms. Good luck.

If you are not of normal weight, odds are your child may not be of normal weight either. When Mom and Dad are overweight, usually the children are overweight. A significant number of children are overweight or obese today. Many have the start of heart disease, and unfortunately, a significant number have type 2 diabetes. Type 2 diabetes is caused by obesity. A very serious problem that can lead to many diseases at a young age. That child will not have a normal life span. In 20 years many will have serious diseases, heart attacks, strokes, blindness and amputations of their extremities—a completely avoidable problem by eating the right food. This needs to be taught at a very young age. Remember I said: it's the mother most of the time, because she's the one buying the food, eighty percent of the time. Gently telling a child what not to eat may not work out. Just buy the right food, and they will get hungry soon enough. Teaching them about avoiding bad food at school is important. Read my book, *The Secret of the Non-diet for Children*, and it will give you some basic education about proper eating..

You need to know your own and you child's BMI. That will tell you whether you are off-track. If your doctor does not check your child's waistline and BMI, maybe you need to find a new doctor. Look at the doctor himself. If he's not in shape, I suspect he will probably not motivate you.

My book recommends low-glycemic complex carbohydrates, whole grain, vegetables and fruit, essentially all-you-can-eat, no diet, just high nutrient dense foods. I don't recommend eating a lot of meat, because is full of cholesterol and fat. If you eat the way I describe, about 80% of the time you'll be of normal weight and have few illnesses in your lifetime, and probably lived to be a hundred, healthy and intelligent. A combination of proper eating and exercise controls stress and a purpose in your life will greatly enhance your chances of achieving that goal.

The motivation of your child will be determined, mostly by what you teach them by your example, and about 30% will be determined by the child itself. The social setting your child grows up in has the greatest effect on what will happen to your children. It takes a community, but parents are most important. All of it should help. I love motivating a children that speak two languages. Most are from economically deprived areas.

How can we make a commitment to change our life towards health and wellness? How can we improve the odds of this being a permanent change?

The desire for consistency is a big motivational factor. Consistency is well founded in psychology. It is this tendency to be consistent, really strong enough to compel us to do what we ordinarily might not do? There is no question about it; consistency has a lot of leg and lifting power. The drive to be consistent constitutes a highly potent weapon of social influence, often causing us to act in ways that are very contrary to our own best interest. We should recognize that in most circumstances, consistency is valued and adaptive. Inconsistency is commonly thought to be an undesirable personality trait.

The person who makes a commitment and whose beliefs, words, and dates don't match their action is seen as two-faced, confused, or even mentally ill. On the other side, a high degree of consistency is normally associated with personal and intellectual strength. He has a strong mind being able to stop smoking. He had a weak mind because he could not stop smoking. That's the kind of thing you hear quite commonly. Personally, unfortunately, I've always thought smokers were a bit weak-minded and I think most all society looks at it that way. Unfortunate but true. Consistency is the heart of logic, rationality, stability and honesty. Sometimes, consistency is valued even more than being right. You may be on the wrong side of an argument, but if you're consistent, you may still be respected.

Good personal consistency is highly valued in our culture. Most of the time we would be better off in our approach to things if it is well laced with consistency. Without it our lives would be difficult.

If you write down your commitment to wellness, losing weight, stopping smoking, taking drugs, look at the statement daily and visualize your commitment, you will be much more likely to achieve your goal, because it is consistent with your thought process.

It is even more likely to happen in the long run if you put it on business cards and then handed them out to a large number of friends, really committing yourself publicly. Because consistency is a basic mental process in our brains, based even on evolution, consistent people are more likely to survive the evolutionary process. I believe it is in our genetic DNA.

Public declaration of your intentions is motivating and more likely to make it happen. Frankly, it would be embarrassing not to carry out your commitment after public declaration. Consistency can become automatic and thoughtless, making it easier to change behavior permanently. Sometimes, though, it may cause you to buy a car or something of that nature because the salesman, using the advantage of the consistency principle, tricks you into saying something and, out of consistency, you buy the car when you didn't really want. It is a well-known sales technique.

It appears automatic consistency functions against thought—you don't have to think. If you try to change something, certainly it's great, but if someone tries to sell you something and you don't want it, it may not be the best. So you need to learn to understand. You have to learn to watch your words on the phone or in the sales room. How is that force engaged? What produces the effect that activates the powerful consistency principle? How do you take advantage of this principle? How do you activate it? Make a commitment. Take a stand. Go on the record. It sets the stage for you automatically with early statements. Professionals of nearly every sort aim commitment statements at us. Their strategies are intended to get you to change and to commit to change. They may ask you to sign a statement.

Sometimes increasing the commitment is motivating. Once you have agreed to the request, your attitude may change; you may become the kind of person who does this sort of thing and develops new habits.

Small requests or trivial requests can influence our self-concepts. It may increase our own compliance. You can use small commitments to manipulate a person's self-image. A step in the right direction can be turned into a bigger commitment. The steps need to be active, public, effortful, and freely chosen. Steps change attitudes and perceptions.

People's true feelings and beliefs are expressed less by their words than their deeds. Character is a sum of your deeds. The rippling impact of behavior is the seed that projects future behavior. A written statement has tremendous power. Set a goal and write it down; read it every day. Put signs on your refrigerator. If hunger is not what you have, food is not what you need. When you have set a goal, you have something for which to aim. There is something magical about writing things down. When you read your goal it will stimulate you.

You're more likely to live up to your statement when you write it down. Written statements are especially effective when they are made public statements. There is an evolutionary genetic drive to activate the stand taken. Personal consistency is a genetic trait and can be counted on to lead you to your stated goal. Public statements can be awesome and get results. Written commitments are most effective in changing a person's self-image and future behavior, especially when they are active, public, and effortful. A commitment must grow its own legs, something to stand on, to assure that the change lasts long-term.

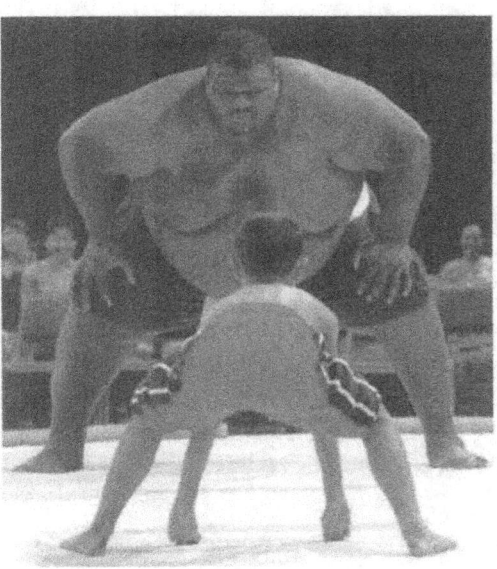

You're losing weight, feeling better, and now you're even starting to look better, but you're not yet at your desired BMI. But, because of the changes, you now have legs to stand on and are now more likely to achieve your goal to be cured of type 2 diabetes by losing the appropriate weight. Type 2 diabetes can be cured 90% of the time if you develop a normal BMI. You're starting to see things differently and this will help in achieving your goal.

It has long been recognized that most people have a desire to act consistently with their beliefs, attitudes, words and deeds. It is valued by society, and fits your public image, and results in some control of your contract and provides a lot of beneficial attributes to your life. It also improves your existence on this earth, and you will probably have a long healthy life. The initial commitment is the key. Committing yourself can cause the growth of legs on your statement and can result in achieving your goal. Consistency in our decisions can be influenced by our own emotions. How we think is everything. Our emotions speak to the whole body through neuropeptides, hormones and neurotransmitters. Your brain speaks to your 70 trillion body cells; your 70 trillion body cells speak to your brain. Your thoughts will control your destiny. Some commonly found traits of commitment include those who are committed to keep their promises. They do what they say long after the moment they said it has passed. People who are committed are in it for the long haul. They are willing to exchange short-term luxuries for a brighter future.

People who are committed have their eye on the finish line, but enjoy the ride there. People who are committed demonstrate a minute-after-minute, day-after-day, month-after-month, and year-after-year attention to ensuring that "mundane" tasks are accomplished, because they know that excellence isn't in the details, it is the details. People who are committed don't build walls; they learn how to surpass them.

Reading a book, attending a lecture, listening to educational CDs, talking to an expert in the field, M.D., or Ph.D. are all ways that can motivate us. There is a genetic tendency in us to listen and follow the recommendations of an authority figure.

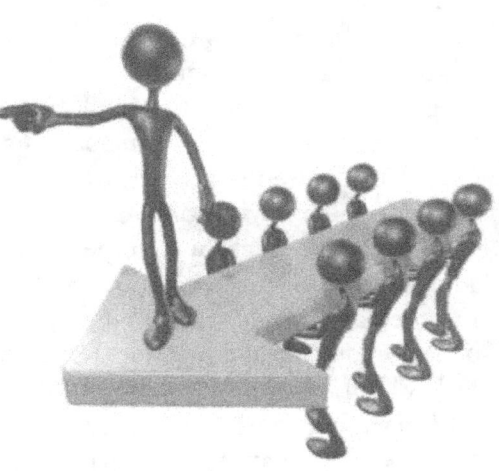

We have a deep-seated sense of duty to authority. This has been studied scientifically. It is the extreme willingness of adults to go to almost any lengths on the command of an authority that constitutes the chief findings of a scientific study. Doesn't that make you wonder about what happened in Germany in the '30s and '40s? Authority was obeyed without question at that time in history, which led to war and the Holocaust.

So "authority" can lead to good, improving your life, health job, and relationships, but also to an extreme. As we see in terroristic acts today, largely related to extreme positions in religion, faith, brainwashing, and to the point of suicide in the name of a cause. So the authority you pick and believe in is critical.

The appearance of authority can be enough. We are often vulnerable to the symbols of authority. Just the symbol of M.D., Ph.D., or a uniform increases their believability, and we are more likely to obey them. Several symbols can reliably trigger our compliance in the absence of any clear knowledge of that authority person. Con artists drape themselves with the symbols of authority. They drive up in a fancy car, fancy clothes, college degrees they don't have and are smooth talkers. They know they are adorned by the principal of authority compliance on our part.

There's no question the size of the authority figure can make a difference. It's in our genetic code. Look at animal behavior, who's in charge of their tribe? The big guy.

In my own experience, as soon as I could afford them. I've always dressed in a nice suit, ties and shoes and drove a fancy car. Believe me, it improved my credibility and ability to motivate my patients to wellness. I'm a surgeon, but I tell you two thirds of my time I spend talking to patients, trying to get them to motivate toward wellness, weight loss, stress reduction, and exercise. There's no question, I spend two thirds of my time teaching patients. It thrills me to know that I can get all the patients well with the word and not the knife. If I can motivate them it will work.

We have a click; whir type of responding and people will take advantage of it. We stop thinking when an authority figure talks to us. But the good part is, if this is their authority, it causes us to change our behavior, quickly and motivate toward wellness. Maybe buying the CD or DVD of an authority you like can reinforce your daily and result in long-term improvement of your health, physically and mentally.

The white coat of a physician, or a nice suit is very significant. More authority than the out-of-shape, poorly dressed, unloving healthcare provider. Your doctor needs to be a placebo; you need to believe in his healing power. If the healthcare provider is not following his recommendations to you, I suspect he will not be a good motivator for you.

People calmly ask me, do I follow the recommendations of my book, *The Secret of the Nondiet*, which I teach? You can is look at me and it's quite obvious that I do. It's motivating to the people I'm speaking to. If I weighed 230 pounds, you think they would listen to me? It would not be motivating.

If the authority figure drives a fancy car, it can have an effect on his authority, pro or con. We need to have a heightened awareness of the authenticity of the provider were listening to. Is the authority sincere, honest, and does he have your best interests at heart? Don't follow the authority to the grave. You know from reading the newspaper that that happens periodically. The Germans followed a powerful figure to the Holocaust. Is the authority truly an expert? Are his degrees real?

There is a genetic component in our mind and strong pressure from society to comply with requests of authority. The strength of this tendency to obey legitimizes the authority. It comes from systematic social practices designed and instilled in us from childhood. It implies obedience, constitutes correct conduct, right or wrong. It can lead to the good and the bad. Sometimes we respond to authority automatically. It is much more likely to happen when the authority has all the symbols, the degrees, the uniform, the stature, the fancy car, the supporting people and perhaps even CDs, DVDs and books. We accord such a person more deference and obedience upon the first encounter. You have to separate faith from facts. That can be very difficult.

HOPE, HOPELESSNESS AND OPTIMISM

These three can all be motivating. How so? Hopelessness
especially would seem to be a dead
end street, but not so. AA, Alco-
holic's Anonymous, uses it as a basic
tenet of its work. It's the motivating
factor.

The 12 steps have a spiritually
motivating factor. Remember,
spirituality and religion are
motivating. Attending religious
services is the path to spirituality.
We are all motivated differently—
different things work for different
people. We've spoken a number
time before about it: don't admit

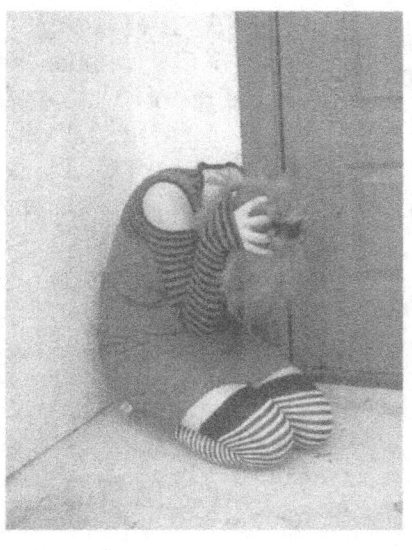

defeat. Then again, for some advanced addictions hopelessness and
defeat seem to be the bottom and we can finally ask for help, admit our
imperfections, and start looking straight up for help. No one likes to
admit defeat. Every natural instinct, all survival, cries out against
powerlessness. Destructive thinking has warped our minds so that only
an act of prominence can remove the plague from us. At AA they
believed that only through utter defeat are we able to take our first steps
toward change.

The admission of personal powerlessness finally turns out to be the
firm bedrock upon which happy and purposeful lives may be rebuilt.
Until you humble yourself, sobriety will be precarious. AA has an
extensive history of having extensive success, but clearly, not for
everyone. There clearly have been failures. The mental obsession of
alcohol is so powerful to some people that no amount of personal
willpower can break it. They have found a belief in spirituality or God
helps tremendously.

The 12 Steps

Step one: We admitted we were powerless over alcohol—that our lives have become unmanageable.

Step two: Came to believe that a power greater than ourselves could restore us to sanity.

Step three: Made a decision to turn our will and our lives over to the care of God, as we understand him.

Step four: Made a searching and fearless moral inventory of ourselves.

Step five: Admitted to God, to ourselves, and to another human being the exact nature of our wrongs.

Step six: Were entirely ready to have God remove all these defects of character.

Step seven: Only ask him to remove our shortcomings.

Step eight: Made a list of all persons we had harmed and became willing to make amends to them all.

Step nine: Major amends to such people wherever possible, except when doing so would injure others.

Step 10: Continue to take personal inventory, and when we were wrong promptly admitted it.

Step 11: Sought through prayer and meditation to improve our conscious contact with God, as we understood him, praying only for knowledge of his will for us and the power to carry that out.

Step 12: Having had a spiritual awakening as a result of the steps, we tried to carry this message to alcoholics, and to practice these principles in all our affairs.

Hope motivates the neuropeptides, hormones and neurotransmitters, all of your brain's actions. It has been proven through scientific studies that people with hope increase their chances of getting better. Pessimism, cancer doctors say, shortens the life span of their patients by as much as 50% and reduces the spontaneous cure rate of cancer. Dr. LaShan, who treated the psychiatric aspect of terminal cancer patients in New York for 45 years, proved that in his scientific studies of his patients. Hope heals, pessimism kills. I have seen it in my patients many times. I have taught many of my cancer patient's mind-body techniques. Their longevity and their hopefulness improved greatly.

When I was a child I lived in New York City, just down the street from where Dr. LaShan practiced medicine. I never met him, but I found it very interesting as to what he did. He took one of his metastatic breast cancer patients to lunch once a month at the Metropolitan Museum of art, which was three blocks from my house. Then he would walk her through the museum for one half hour, looking at her favorite art. This was the office visit. He did this for five years. When she was restudied after five years, there was no trace of cancer. He clearly cured her with hope and visualization techniques. I would have loved to meet that man.

I recently had a young man with metastatic lung cancer from smoking with a two tumors the size of tennis balls clearly visible in his neck. Around October I asked him to visualize a Pac Man coming in and eating up his tumor, a chemical coming in and eating the tumor and to visualize he was urinating it out of his body. Then I asked him to meet me on July 4 at noon on my pier at Lake Wawasee for lunch. I knew he fished that lake a lot and knew where my pier was. He showed up at noon with four fish on a stringer. He said he caught them under my pier earlier in the day. Promoting hope and visualization can remind the body what it is like to be well and affect your immunity. Clearly the neuropeptides and hormones, and neurotransmitters of hope are destroying his cancer.

My son is a neurosurgeon. He came to me one day and said, "I think I know what you're talking about now." His patient was a woman with four children and no husband and it looked like she had a very small highly malignant tumor on her MRI scan. He told her it looked malignant. She asked how long she had to live. He said six to nine months and gave her a small amount of hope. She started screaming and it lasted all night. The next day he did a biopsy, which proved the point, and again told her she had six to nine months to live. Unfortunately, this patient with a very small malignant tumor was dead the next day. Having no hope caused her hopelessness.

People who have hope set high goals for themselves. Then neurotransmitters, neuropeptides, hormones, heal them by affecting their own immunity.

Hope plays a potent role in life. Hope is more than a sunny view that events will turn out all right. It's motivating. It says that you believe, that you have the will and the way to accomplish your goals.

People tend to have differences in the degree to which they have hope based on their lives. Some typically see themselves as able to get out of a jam or find a way to solve the problem, while others do not see themselves as having the energy, ability, or means to accomplish their goals. People with increased levels of hope have certain traits, among them being able to motivate themselves, feeling resourceful enough to find ways to cope. Their objectives: reassuring themselves, being flexible, finding different ways to get to the goals or to switch goals, or break things down into smaller tasks, they can accomplish a little bit at a time. They express emotional intelligence. Having hope means one will not give in to overwhelming anxiety, an attitude of depression in the face of difficult, challenging times. People who are hopeful have less depression. Depression slows you down you find yourself tired all day.

Optimism is a great motivator and a close friend or relative of hope. Optimism, like hope, means having a strong expectation that bad things will turn out all right in life, despite setbacks and frustrations. Optimism is an attitude that buffers people; it prevents falling into apathy, hopelessness, or depression in the face of tough going. And, as with hope, its near cousin, optimism pays dividends in life. Of course it means you must be realistic in your optimism. I don't dream to be an NBA basketball player, but I hope to be the national 85-and-over tennis champ in 12 years. It's possible. I train for it every day. Optimism defines how people explain success and failure to themselves. Optimists see failure as something that can be changed; so then they can succeed the next time. Pessimists take the blame for failure, ascribing it to some hopeless condition they cannot change.

Optimism predicts success in health habits and basic living. The emotional reaction to defeat is crucial to the ability to marshal enough motivation to continue or to prove yourself.

A positive or negative outlook may well be inborn in some people. Some people are just plain optimists and others pessimistic all their lives. My dad read the New York Daily News every day. No wonder he was generally a pessimistic person, in spite of his only son never giving him trouble and became a well-known neurosurgeon and provided a beautiful home for his mom and dad and a place in Florida to stay in the wintertime. Newspapers have in them only bad news. I don't think he ever realized that.

Optimism and hope—like helplessness and despair—can be learned. Underlying both is an outlook that psychologists call self-efficacy—the belief that one has mastery over the events of one's life and can meet the changing challenges. Peoples' beliefs about their abilities have a profound effect; they can be liabilities or assets. Pick your path!

Chi-gung is the Asian way of mindfulness, paying more attention to how we think. It has great motivating benefits for healing and wellness. It's a way of life leading to longer changes in the thinking process and leads to great results.

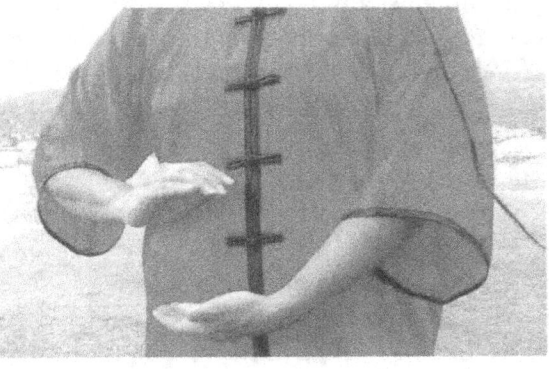

Chi-gung is an ancient Chinese system of self-cultivation developed specifically as a means by which each individual may take full responsibility for protecting health, promoting vitality, and prolonging life, while cultivating spiritual awareness and insight. Based on the primordial principles of classical Taoist philosophy, chi-gung is simple and practical. It's motivating to self-improvement, wellness, work, and spirituality. The practitioner learns how to harness the fundamental forces of the cosmos and balances them with the elemental energies of nature and harmonizes them both with the essence, energy and spirit (the three treasures of human life). Chi-gung thus enables the individual to amplify his or her personal power with the infinite power of the universe.

Known in traditional Chinese thought, as the "three powers", heaven, earth and humanity represent the sum total of all the forces in factors at all levels of human existence within the universe as we know it. It is by virtue of the balance and harmony of the powers that we may enjoy health and vitality, attain power and longevity, enhance our mental awareness and spiritual insight, and realize the primordial immortality of the human spirit.

Chi means breath and air and, by extension, denotes energy and vitality. Gung is a general term meaning the work. Chi-Gung may be translated as breath exercise as well as energy work. It is slow poetic body movements. When you read about Chinese and Asian medical care, acupuncture, chi-gung, they talk about your chi—too little, too much—moving about your body. Energy and movement, everything in this world is energy and vibration. That goes back 5000 years. When you're in China, you will see them doing it outside the hotel every morning. At any age, Chi constitutes the dynamic for field in which all energy moves and from which all power springs. Every type of energy functions with in its own specific force field.

Chi-Gung involves various degrees of gentler movement or stillness of the body, balanced with rhythmical regular breathing, with a calm, unhurried and clearly focused mind. Soft slow movement of the body prevents the stiffness and stagnation that lead to degeneration and death.

These slow movements, with mindfulness, are considered meditation, because they blend soft gentle movements of the body with a calm contemplative state of mind. In the moving forms of chi-gung, the external motions of the body need to be coordinated with the main body.

The original meaning of the Chinese "the Tao" is "the way"—a way of life. That is why doing chi-gung can motivate you to a healthy life, throw off bad habits, whether it be eating, lack of exercise, alcohol, cigarettes or drugs, anxiety or depression. You become more mindful and consider the consequences of your actions. You can learn about chi-gung through books, DVDs, personal instruction, or class at my yoga institute, Anytime Fitness, or the local Y. if you do this regularly, certainly it will lead to wellness.

MOTIVATION AND TAI CHI

Tai chi is a sequence of slow, meditative movements, a hybrid of yoga and martial arts, based on the cyclical movements of the natural world. Tai chi promises us a more harmonious connection to our familiar routines, to reconnect us to the ground for energy that permeates the entire universe. When that energy becomes truly available to us, our vitality is boundless.

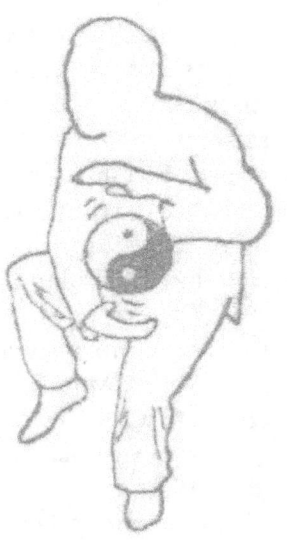

It is a great physical and mental process to promote wellness in our lives. It helps bring serenity to our mind and health to our body. A great way to give up bad habits: removing the need for them. Tai chi increases dopamine, the feel-good chemical in our brain—a substitute for alcohol drugs and cigarettes, and a much more healthy approach.

In Chinese, tai chi literally means "infinity". Tai chi is a gentle yet effective path to allowing that healing energy to flow freely. The study of tai chi allows a student a combined grace and tranquility of the body. It allows the student to experience the interplay of yin and yang energies. They create harmonious rhythms that animate the natural world.

The principal or philosophy of tai chi started over 10,000 years ago. The people in China began to closely observe the cycles of nature, eventually developing a series of movements based on the dynamic patterns of the natural world. Tai chi is one of the most popular of these systems of self awareness and physical development. Based on the recognition that our bodies are like miniature universes, the gentle movements of tai chi helps our inner energy flow like the flow of nature itself. We've got to keep moving.

Feeling how energy circulates through our bodies with the movements of tai chi, we become intimate with the laws of the universe. Doing tai chi means balancing ourselves physically, emotionally, and spiritually. In tai chi, we move, but gently enough to preserve inner calm and composure. The subtle energy of our mind and spirit merges with the coarser energy of our body.

In tai chi, we are not merely striving to achieve precise physical movements. We are learning the secrets of physical health and longevity by participating in the cycles of energy that flow through the universe. All life consists of cycles, even the energies of organisms that circulate through the body. When you look at the sky and the universe, you notice everything is organized, essentially, in a circular pattern. Tai chi teaches us to transform a straight line of energy into a circle, putting us in touch with a never-ending energy. Everything in the universe tends to follow a circular pattern. The Earth spins on its axis as it orbits the sun. The sun, in turn, orbits the galactic center of the Milky Way. The galaxy itself forms a circular pattern as it courses through the universe. All of the movements of tai chi are a series of circles, which reflect this cosmic law.

As this primal chi energy moves, it has a polarizing effect: yin and yang, light and dark, feminine and masculine, left and right, and so on. The dynamic interaction of these polarities accounts for the endless variety of the physical world, which, for all its diversity, is still fundamentally one. Through our practice of tai chi, we gain official knowledge of this unity amidst diversity.

The practice of tai chi trains a mind to observe the body in every detail. In this way, rather than scattering energies through mindless physical activity, we gather and retrain it. The peaceful mental atmosphere created by tai chi movement helps negative thought patterns to dissolve and be replaced by positive, life-enhancing attitudes. Tai chi accomplishes this without dogma or a rigid belief system. It improves the personalities by refining and harmonizing our yin and yang energies, resulting in an even temperament and calm disposition. These qualities enable us to remain poised even in the most difficult situations. After all, to be excessively positive or negative is ultimately madness. Only by harmonizing the dualities in a mind can we achieve the balance that brings us peace.

What is chi? Chi energy circulates continuously through the channels of our bodies, not unlike the water flows in a riverbed. But most people's chi is weak, pooled and stagnating in cavities instead of powerfully flowing. Minds can influence the circulation of chi. The more we train our minds and our chi the more responsive and powerful they become. Accordingly, when the mind and chi are in concert, we enjoyed harmony and health. When the mind and chi are at cross purposes, it is chaos and disease. In tai chi we learn movements that both contract and expand chi energy. This flow of chi is the dance of yin and yang. Tai chi is a moving meditation. Tai chi trains a body and mind to function as one. It fosters calm and self-control, even during times of extreme duress. Those who pursue tai chi as a martial art find that it helps them to defend themselves in a controlled and balanced manner without fear or anger. Even those who practice tai chi simply for health find it useful when they are called upon to defend themselves. The majority of people do tai chi to establish confidence and physical control.

Tai chi has many healing benefits and is a great practice for wellness. I know of no one that practices tai chi regularly who is not on a wellness path. Tai chi is a self-healing practice that can be enjoyed by anyone, regardless of age, fitness, or state of health. No matter what your physical condition, your weight or your disability, we can teach you tai chi. Consistent practice of tai chi balances our internal energy so effectively that it has been known to alleviate or even cure a wide variety of ailments, including high blood pressure, arthritis, ulcers, tuberculosis, heart disease, and chronic pain. It helps us avoid disease by keeping our internal energies in a state of balance. When our energy becomes blocked or impeded, we get sick. Disease tells us our energy flow needs to be adjusted. Tai chi helps us to release the vitality locked within our tense and anxious bodies. Many of us hope for long life, but we want to live to be vigorous, healthy and happy, even in old age. We also know that having a tranquil spirit plays a crucial role in helping us to endure the often troubled and troubling world. Given the pace of modern life, we can grow old very fast. Tai chi offers us a strategy for achieving that not only calmness but also rejuvenation. I practice it nightly and feel like I control my mind and body.

OUR FRONTAL LOBE IS IN CHARGE AND MOTIVATES US

One way or another, we are the ones who will make the decision on what to eat. We are the authors of our own health. We are the driver of that tank that is involved with this war of eating.

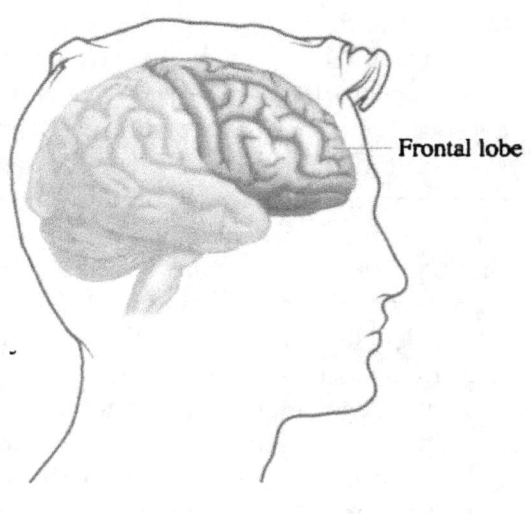

Frontal lobe

Women have more eating problems than men because they are in charge more of the meal preparation, buying the food, and a constant barrage from the media and magazines about body size.

Can you imagine buying food for a husband, yourself, and the children who all have different appetites and food preferences, and she is trying to control the situation. The husband may have the "inflexible palate syndrome" and just will not change what he eats in spite of being a diabetic or heart patient. The husband says. "I can't possibly live without eating meat every day." The children are screaming out for sugary, fatty and salty foods.

I would say with children it's a bit easier, because they will get hungry and you are buying the food. If there is a problem and your children are overweight, have an honest look at them. Don't deny the picture, bring in changes slowly, and they may not notice it. Their tastes buds will change. I slowly introduced a lot of vegetarian food at the doctors' lounge in the hospital. Frankly, they did not notice it and the food looks great now. The dietitian is a friend of mine. Next week she's bringing in edamame on a regular basis. Sooner or later, the children's tastes buds will change. Educate them about school food, to read labels, to avoid sugary drinks. The husband could be more of a problem. He may need to be educated about healthy food. Believe me, in my 45 years of being a physician; Americans in general eat the mad, toxic, sad foods, all fat, sugar, and salt. The killer triad of Americans.

Limiting your own or family members food intake is like a starvation diet; it will not work and will result in over eating and snacking. When preparing food yourself on a daily basis. It makes it a lot more difficult, and quite easy to feed your own psychology with food. The food that causes the flow of dopamine is in your hand, a very tempting situation. Besides, you may be hungry. You look at food every day, making the meals and testing your self-control daily and sometimes multiple times a day. It is difficult for many. Family members may use food to control each other socially. One never eats; another over eats. One is perfect, and another is out of control. Being overweight, people think you're out of control, that you have emotional problems. Thinness is considered being in control, but many times it is not.

Society looks at people with a normal weight as being in control of their lives. Social stigma is related to body size.

Eating control was thought to be the solution to obesity, when the answer to me is much more the type of food you are eating. Control will follow that if you're eating the correct food. If you are eating a high nutrient dense food pattern, in general, you do not need to watch even your portions. Most of the time, it is difficult for us to have perfect control of our eating habits. I say, "food selection" should lead the way to good health and proper weight.

Over-controlling behavior with food is a central problem with eating disorders, anorexia and bulimia.

You'll get some families, like I saw last week, gathered around the table at a Japanese restaurant, where I clearly saw them all, twenty feet in front of me, from three-year-olds to 80-year-olds, about 10 of them, all seriously overweight. Children with puffy cheeks, adults with bellies hanging down, men and women. It was a sad sight. I would say odds are they a totally blind to their situation. Just like an anorexic.

How did this happen? Genetics, accounts for only 20%. Probably they're like the anorexic, and many overweight people, they don't see it in themselves. You do not see the potential health problems, and that is frankly all I'm talking about. I don't care about the cosmetics; many of these people are beautiful. I passionately care about their future of diabetes, heart disease and strokes, arthritis, dementia and cancer. Their psychiatric needs and eating behavior probably are the same throughout the family; the anxiety and probably the lack of serotonin to feel good are about the same. Instead of a tranquilizer, they are using food to feel good. They have a similar way of cooking, same type of food, most likely lack of proper eating education. I would bet two or three already have diabetes, maybe one of them even as a teenager. I would bet everything I own that the two or three diabetics do not know that their type 2 diabetes is curable by getting down to a normal weight.

Food preferences are transmitted within the family from parent to child. Pleasurable fatty food, and sugary food, chemically decreases anxiety, increases love. It's the womb, that caves, and escape from life's problems. The poor have this need, of course, more commonly. That is the reason they have a much higher rate of overweight and obesity. It's their only daily pleasure, many times. There is much more obesity in the economically distressed. Food is also used among family members to distribute power, rewards, and to control behavior. Eating behavior is used many times among family members to assume power and control.

Eating behavior can keep the family together: the hell with the rest of the world, this is us! An individual's thoughts and beliefs and attitudes greatly affect what they eat. Many people justify their food choices with incorrect information they obtain from some ineffective diet book. Many of the diet books are complete frauds. Individuals have a range of beliefs about the meaning of food system, body size and shape. Many believe diets are all or nothing and give up too easily.

Food deprivation will lead to overeating. High-protein diets don't work. Starving yourself of carbohydrates will sooner or later lead to overeating. Negative beliefs about obesity may motivate some people to a normal weight—I don't want to look this way—and they become motivated to change. It's a complex psychological situation between the pleasure of eating and subsequent guilt.

As we know women are the main providers of food in the family. Gender is central to many of the conflicts surrounding food. Eighty percent of the clients in my eating classes are female. There are a number of reasons for that, as we already know, including self-image, and being overweight is more common in general among women. They also choose education about proper eating more commonly. Men don't want to give up that steak and would rather exercise. Women are treated differently in the media. You have to be thin to be on TV, although we have witnessed the yo-yo diets of Oprah. I suspect that situation is all about psychology. Women show more body dissatisfaction than men, and also body size is more important to women's self-esteem.

Most of the anorexics and bulimics are women. Abdominal fat is more dangerous, and men have more of that, female fat is usually around the buttocks and thighs.

Food choice is affected by social norms. Certain ethnic groups make better or worse, food choices. The famous China study by Dr. Colin Campbell, where they studied Chinese people and related eating patterns. In other cultures, overweight and obesity is rampant in more than 50% of the people, and those cultures have diabetes and its consequences. Family and cultural norms affect our image of ourselves. Certain ethnic groups accept obesity.

Dieting, not food selection is a media choice to lose weight. Which sells diet books, but they usually don't work. They're not concerned since they already made the money.

Social norms of attractiveness, contribute to the discrimination and stereotypes of being overweight and obese. Peer influence and social support can be used to modify eating behavior in the overweight. And this is a socially desirable state, which can lead to eating disorders. The psychological effects of the chemicals of food—dopamine, serotonin, endorphins, and beta-endorphin—probably are the great drivers of food choices and habits.

The individual, the family, the group, have great effects on the food choices that we make. Some ethnic groups think cheese is everything, although, mind you, it's 80% fat.

We have to eat everyday, so the cue is there continuously, lack of serotonin cries out for relief. It will take a combination of stress relief, exercise and food choice that will lead to proper eating habits and good health. You are the author of your health! Fat, sugar and salt have the nasty chemicals that lead to being overweight and obese. Good luck in your choices.

The Motivation of Placebo and Nocebo

Placebo means to please, nocebo means to harm. A pill, a doctor, and occasionally even a procedure can result in healing if we believe that it will. That's the power of the placebo. The placebo effect can be between 30 to 70%. It depends on our faith in that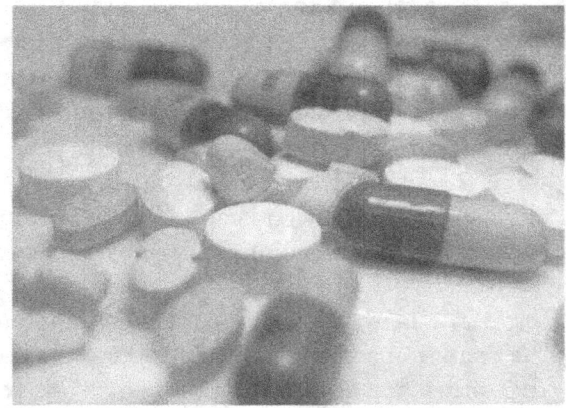
medication, It causes chemical changes in our body and brain and we become well. It's been known about for thousands of years.

So a doctor, a medication and yes, even in operation, which found nothing, can motivate us toward wellness, It's all over the medical literature and in my personal experience in over 40 years of medical practice. The reason I always wear fancy clothes in my office is because it produces confidence in my patients. The patient believes I can get them well. Their chemistry responds and motivates them to get well.

A healthcare provider, overweight, out of shape will have difficulty motivating the patient through the placebo effect. The placebo costs little and is very cheap. And a loving healthcare provider, the occasional hug, the smile, and friendly conversation, beginning with. "What's going on in your life?" can heal the patient.

Recently, I was treating the owner of a company with 35 employees for severe sciatica. I found nothing on the MRI scan, and did not recommend surgery. I tried every measure possible, but he just did not get better. One day he came to me and said, if I did nothing to help him, he would have to close his small factory on Monday and put 35 people out of work. This made the situation even more serious; 35 people could lose their job. I told him I could explore the nerve that I thought was involved with this pain and see if he had a hidden ruptured disk. I operated on him and found nothing. Trying to be a healer, not trying to be his deceitful, I told him I took some pressure off the nerve by removing some arthritic bone, and gave a lot more room to the nerve. The following day, all this pain was gone, and he was back at work on Monday, and so were 35 other people. I think it was the placebo effect of the operation. That can happen. I am sure that surgeons who generally over operate (believe me there are plenty of them) take full of vantage of that. And that patients many times are better for a few months through the placebo effect. You can see a placebo can be motivating in itself. Because of your belief in what is done, or the pill or the healthcare provider, faith causes chemical changes in the body and can motivate you to wellness.

The nocebo can motivate you toward unnecessary procedures. The healthcare provider takes advantage of modern technology, like CT scans, MRIs, scoping procedures and angiograms to impress you that the changes on the studies are related to your complaints, when many times they are not, to do a procedure on you. I see this a lot in back surgery, gallbladder surgery, hysterectomies, cosmetic surgery and an occasional heart operation. I have personally experienced that many times in my 40 years of practicing surgery. In essence, the nocebo, the negative speak, is used to promote a procedure. They hand you the CT, MRI, angiographic report, and you carry it around with you convincing you of the seriousness of your problem, when in reality it may not mean very much. That makes it a lot easier for the provider to talk you into something. That's why I called the "nocebo" the evil twin. It can motivate you toward an unnecessary operation or procedure. I've written a book called *Nocebo-Placebo's Evil Twin*. You might enjoy reading it and it may save you an unnecessary procedure. The book can be found on my website *www.kachmannmindbody.com*.

MOTIVATION AND YOGA

Yoga is an excellent way to motivate yourself toward wellness. It's about the body and the mind. It connects the mind to the body, the body to the mind. Although I am a full-time neurosurgeon, I own two wellness studios. It helps my patients and me a great deal.

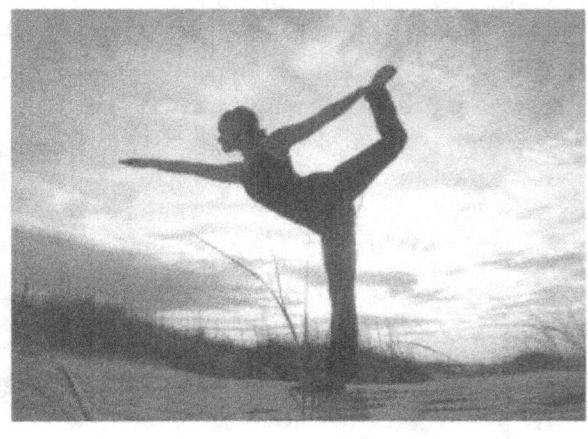

Yoga is a science, not a religion, the focus of which is you and me and how we relate to the universe around us. If the pressures of today's world leave you feeling frazzled and out of sorts, practicing the science of yoga can help you feel whole again. Yoga's techniques, which have been discovered and developed through various methods, have been used for thousands of years to address mental, emotional and spiritual conflicts.

The study of yoga dates back 5000 years. It is now spreading throughout the Western world and is practiced extensively in every city in the United States. Yoga has withstood the test of time.

Yoga is a Sanskrit word, most commonly translated as "union," "yoking," or "bringing together." Sanskrit words not only have intellectual meaning, they also have a deeper resonance. For instance, Ohm, the background sound of the universe, is said to include all sounds at once. And, therefore, all knowledge, all potential, all inspiration—in short, all things at once.

Sanskrit existed first as a language of sound. The relative simplicity of Sanskrit made it easier for early practitioners to pass on orally the knowledge of yoga. It was years later that written characters came into existence. The oldest written records of yoga—the Vedas, yoga Sutras, the Hatha Yoga and other ancient writings, are in Sanskrit. Nowadays knowledge of Sanskrit is not necessary to begin the practice of yoga.

Yoga is a state of oneness realized once one has stopped the fluctuations of the mind. This happens when, through disciplined practice, one is free of thoughts, limitations, and distractions, and one can experience for extended periods of time the uninterrupted state of oneness with all things, called samadhi. As everyone is able to practice yoga, everyone has the potential to experience that state of samadhi.

Most commonly, yoga is regarded as a physical discipline. A physical yoga practice consists of exercises called postures, or asana, that strengthen, stretch and outline the body. The brilliance of an asana practice lies in its mindful execution, not in how far you can go in each pose. Each asana requires harnessing together the body and the breath.

After practicing a handful of poses with care and conscious awareness, you'll be transported away from your troubles and feelings of fatigue and begin to feel energized and refreshed—a very motivating way to begin the day. Reduced stress and more energy. The asanas not only condition the body's exterior, but they also work wonders inside the body. The benefits of physical practice include long lean muscles, correct posture, improved breathing and digestion, better circulation, a relaxed nervous system, and fortified immune system. The various postures create an internal massage of the organs, tissues, and muscles; prevent atrophy that results from disuse; and release the tension caused by overexertion or misuse of the muscles.

They are literally thousands of asanas you can learn. They are performed, so the prospect of being bored by yoga is remote. The asanas can be performed in a rigorous fashion, creating a tremendous amount of heat and sweat, or for a change of pace your approach can be much more gentle and soothing. A sequence of postures can be performed in a style that flows from the breath and focuses less on form, or a pose can be held statically, with an eye to the minutest of details. A physical practice can be adapted to whatever the student requires. Age, body type, strength, flexibility, or current or past medical history, need not prevent someone from enjoying the benefits of yoga. Group classes run in levels from introductory to advanced.

The practicing you'll do is a wonderful complement to other sports activities, so you need not drop everything else you're doing in order to take up yoga. For example, I play a lot of tennis, including tournaments, and yoga helps my concentration and flexibility and strengthens my body. It is an excellent way to treat all medical conditions, including especially chronic pain. The flexibility, total body strength, and clear focus that yoga creates are ideal for running, golf, tennis, biking, swimming, softball, skiing and you name it.

Yoga is a great mental discipline. Practicing the asanas requires an attention to detail that helps develop sharp observation skills. Sitting still and meditating, what future to focus on a single point for an extended period of time, being able to draw the mind inward, away from outside distractions, with clear space in your brain for what's essential. It's a good way to get away from addictions. Studies have shown meditation to be effective in treating an array of disorders, including chronic pain, unexplained infertility, high blood pressure, cardiovascular disease, PMS, and psoriasis. Yoga is meditation. You concentrate on every movement, and that is meditation.

Yoga is an emotional journey. It seeks to bring out the best in a person, the joy that is at the core of every being. You can practice anything you'll do in any group at home by yourself. And each has its own reward. It is quality time spent away from the responsibilities and needs of others. It's a chance for you to relax, rejuvenate, and rebound so that you are ready for whatever surprises life has in store for you. I encourage you to spend at least 15 minutes a day doing yoga, and perhaps join a yoga class at a studio for an hour twice a week. I do it on a regular basis.

Yoga is not religion, but can be a spiritual endeavor. You can develop an expanded awareness of the world around you and a deeper appreciation of who you really are. But a belief in God or a supreme being is not a prerequisite to this journey. And at the same time, there is no harmful confusion if you believe in the existence of a higher creative force. All people, regardless of religious affiliation will benefit from having a healthier body, a clearer mind, and a more complete way of breathing, which is what yoga practice will give you.

There are many different styles of yoga. Hatha yoga is one the most common styles. It means the sun and the moon. It describes the practices used to balance your sun and moon qualities. You learn to stretch the tight areas, strengthen weak areas, and bring balance to the opposite polarity within you, the left and right brain. This style of yoga, you may wish to learn is dependent on what you're reading, watching, or interested in. They are all effective.

AYURVEDA, is a form of Indian medicine involving the ancient practice of Indian healing. AYUR means "life." And veda means "science." It is a yoga of rebalancing your current condition, vikritti, to its unique harmonious constitution, your prakriti. It is an ancient Indian way of healing and has great value.

Yoga is an excellent way to motivate yourself to a life of good physical and mental health. It will open your mind to your true potential and help you commit yourself to a better life.

When you're talking about health, love has a lot to do with it. Let's face it, if you're trying to attract or get the attention of another person, getting in shape and looking good works a lot of the time. If you don't take care of yourself, you certainly are less likely to be found attractive by another individual. Are you overweight? Do you smell like cigarettes? Don't discount the power of love. If you're harboring feelings of anger, anxiety or lack

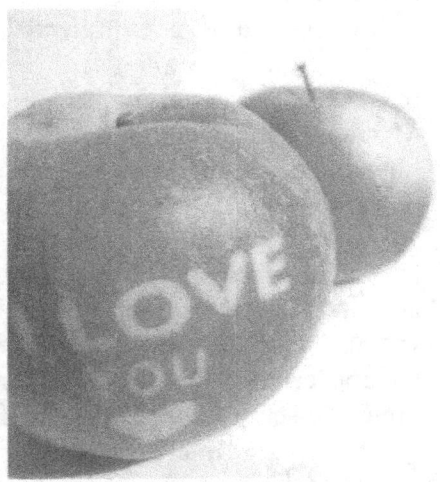

self-esteem, this negative way of thinking could be eating away at your immune system and your health. Your immune system feels what you feel. If your body feels love, it is much more likely to heal. Love of another person, a family, or group can lead to healing. I personally have seen it many times in my 41 years of practicing medicine. Love is a vast and open-ended sensation, the most written about, talked about, and worried about emotion in the history of humankind and can be expressed in countless ways.

Love can be love of nature. It can mean you feel oneness with the universe. It gives us a warm, fuzzy emotion you have been doing something as simple as appreciating a cozy fireplace or watching a movie with your loved one, or the warm sensation when you hug someone. Love is the sense of appreciation, understanding, sympathy, and empathy. It expresses connection, whether it is to a family member or just a friend, or even a perfect stranger.

Love is the antidote to hate, anger, fear and sadness. Your 70 trillion cells feel good when you feel love. Your 70 trillion body cells feel pain when you lead a life without love. Our immune system is very attuned to our feelings.

It has been proved scientifically that negative thinking and emotions accelerate aging and cause heart disease, cancer and inflammatory diseases. Studies published in the American Medical Association Journal.

It is well known that happy people are healthier. Happy people live longer with cancer, and the spontaneous cure rate goes up. That is well publicized in medical literature. If we experienced love of life, the longer we will live and be more protected against a lot of diseases of aging.

Love can be defined as an inner peace, an attitude that can arise from faith, from a spiritual belief system, and the rewards are plentiful. Married people live longer; a person living in isolation has a lot more illness and dies a lot sooner. We all know that, many times after the death of a spouse, the survivor may die within a year or two.

The love of nature has a lot of healing properties. Look what a walk in the park or woods can do for you. It's rejuvenating. I speak to the animals and flowers and find it exhilarating. A walk down a city street will also do that for you. One of the most extraordinary kinds of love is an appreciation for the wonder of nature and for the awesome interconnections between all the facets of the world. Just walking in a quiet rain or early snow can be very rejuvenating. Once when sitting in a tree, observing nature and watching the day go by—I don't hunt—the dew started falling from the leaves, the sun started rising, it was heavenly. Little droplets of water, falling out of the sky, bringing dew on all the grass, plants and trees can get you to fall in love with nature and has many healing properties. How can you not feel love for nature? It can be very motivating to wellness.

There are countless ways to feel love. When you're with someone, it can be a hug, a touch, or look. Just to say "I love you" can be very healing and motivate you to wellness. Interpersonal love heals. Lovers livelonger, that has been scientifically proven. People who are in painful relationships have more illnesses and die sooner and develop bad health habits because of the stress. We all have heard of the broken-heart syndrome "stress cardiomyopathy". Sudden emotional stress can put you in the intensive care unit, be life-threatening, and can cause changes in your EKG, shortness of breath, and even heart failure. Yet, no changes are found on the angiogram. Most of these people do recover. Being in a high-quality relationship has been found to be protective for the heart.

Don't forget to love yourself, which can be most difficult if what you are doing is not consistent with the image of yourself. That's the biggest cause of stress. The inability to cope with threats, real or imaginary, to our emotional, physical, and spiritual being, is the best definition of stress. We all want to be happy, we want to be loved, and we want to love others. That is motivational and healing. Social connectedness improves health and longevity, and social isolation increases mortality. Love is motivating, hate and anger, demotivating. I can clearly tell when treating my patients, by checking the social history—the amount of family love they are exposed to—what the odds of that person healing themselves are. Isolated people don't do well. Let your currency be love and happiness. Be a happy person and say loving things to other people. Leave notes of love around the house, the community around you will send you love in return. That's healing.

Dr. Mark Liponis, the medical director of the Canyon Ranch in Arizona and Massachusetts, calls love vitamin L. He states, often his patients have so much money, freedom, good jobs, fancy homes, but they lack the most important asset—love. I found that recently in a neighbor of mine in Naples Florida. He lives in the fanciest place I ever did see, but I felt sorry for him. He lived there by himself for months at a time, while his wife was back home in Chicago. She went around the world last year by herself on a 747 Jet. How sad, he did not have good health and complained of being lonely. Well, I now have a new friend, who I will be inviting to go to dinner with my wife and me when I get back to Florida next week. With little love in your life, the need for food can be demotivating and not healthy for you. It takes a lifetime of work to be loving, but we can always get better. Even if love is atrophied, it can be revived and renewed, as long as you want to restore it.

Dr. Mark Liponis has a number of recommendations. Tell someone you love him or her, get a pet, keep a love journal, read some books. On page 173 of his book, *Ultra Longevity*, he lists a number of books, you can read. One that he recommends is *The Art of happiness: a Handbook for Living* by the Dalai Lama. He also recommends watching some loving and funny movies, using a love mantra like the one I plan to use, and he recommends "All You Need Is Love" by the Beatles.

Lennon/McCartney

Love, love, love, love, love, love, love, love, love.
There's nothing you can do that can't be done.
Nothing you can sing that can't be sung.
Nothing you can say but you can learn how to play the game
It's easy.

There's nothing you can make that can't be made.
No one you can save that can't be saved.
Nothing you can do but you can learn how to be you
in time - It's easy.

All you need is love, all you need is love,
All you need is love, love, love is all you need.
Love, love, love, love, love, love, love, love, love.
All you need is love, all you need is love,
All you need is love, love, love is all you need.
There's nothing you can know that isn't known.
Nothing you can see that isn't shown.
Nowhere you can be that isn't where you're meant to be.
It's easy.
All you need is love, all you need is love,
All you need is love, love, love is all you need.
All you need is love (all together now)
All you need is love (everybody)
All you need is love, love, love is all you need.

Let's get to work. There can be great benefits and bring love into
your life. It will motivate you to happiness, a long life, a lot of energy,
and very little sickness.

THE BEST OF
DR. RUDY'S MOTIVATION PRINCIPLES

The Rudy in You is a great book about motivation to success in sports by Rudy Ruetigger. You may have seen the movie, which was about building teamwork, fair play and sportsmanship.

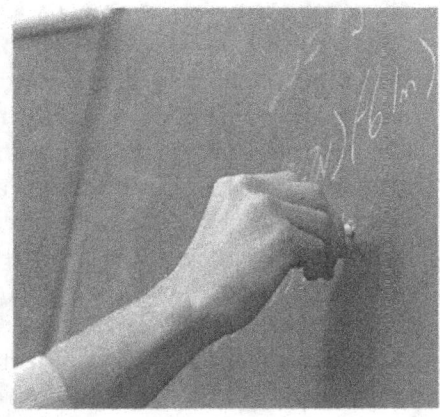

But my name is Rudy too. A lot of the principles laid down by Notre Dame's Rudy are actually what I teach to motivate success and wellness. Of the 40 or so most powerful motivators, I would like to pick the top 10 to my way of thinking.

Before I do that, I would like to tell you my story of my interest in motivation. Recently, I was the guest speaker at a National Chiropractic Association meeting. I gave my talk on reversing type 2 diabetes by eating a proper diet, and a very nice chiropractic doctor stood up and said, "Thank you. The information is great, but how do I motivate my patient to follow it?" I think that's a very fair question, and I decided to read a lot about it and write a book about it, as this information has only limited value if people don't use it to become well.

Why does Dr. Rudy (myself) have such a great interest in the teaching of wellness? For one, all my life I've had a great interest in playing sports of all types. I was not a natural athlete at anything. As a matter of fact, in high school I used to have to try to gain weight. In grade school and high school, I always tried to join a sports team, all the sports. I lived in New York City and played at Central Park every day, handball, tennis, and baseball. I tried very hard to become good at the sports but my ability was limited let's say at best, a little bit above average. My father had no interest in sports. He worked in his delicatessen day and night. Only through a lot of practice, did I get good enough to make the baseball team, basketball team, and, yes, even the football team. I had a lot of help as it was a small school. I weighed only 135 pounds, but playing sports certainly was a good step to wellness. I was not an overweight teenager. My parents consistently ate the wrong deli food, fat, sugary and salty food. They were both overweight.

The teaching of exercise and nutrition was not part of medical school, and it barely is now. I was at my 45th medical school reunion recently and they said, does anyone have any questions. There were three female medical students at luncheon and I asked them how much they had learned about nutrition and wellness. All three said: very little. That was a very sad day for me, and it still has not changed.

After I started my practice and looked closely at my patient's medical problems, remember I'm a neurosurgeon; I developed a sense early in my practice that the majority of illnesses and diseases I was looking at were self-inflicted. Stress, lack of exercise, and what the patients were eating was a cause of 50 to 80% of what I was treating. Many were type 2 diabetics from being overweight. That could be simply corrected by being the proper weight. Then I found a book, *How to Live 365 Days a Year*, by Dr. Schindler. I handed out about 5000 copies free to my patients. They took about $3000 off my quarterly bonuses to pay for it by my corporation. And I was happy to do it. A lot of patients get well without injections, medications or surgery. I felt like I was a doctor doing what was right. After all, the word physician means teacher. We are not graduating teachers from the medical school.

Eventually I read everything I could get my hands on about wellness and found out that, frankly, it's all interrelated and my knowledge base grew tremendously. My motivation to teach this on a wider scale flew off the charts. I don't seem to be able to keep quiet about it, no matter where I go. I now have a wellness center with a yoga studio. We teach proper eating, exercise, individual and group training, meditation, stress reduction, dancing and many other programs. My website is *www.KachmannMindBody.com*. By December I will probably have 10 published books, all in every aspect of wellness. I formed the Mind-Body Index, a list of illnesses caused partially or totally by the mind, usually stress. I made about 20 CDs and DVDs, one-hour lectures on the effects of the aspect of the mind on the human body, about stress, cancer, exercise, proper eating, the nocebo effect, etc. I give at least 30 lectures a year on wellness and have a one-hour weekly TV show about wellness that attracts a large audience.

Clearly, it was a love of teaching the patient how to get well without having to give him dangerous medications or doing surgery that inspired me. Really, it's about the love for the patient, the ability to make them well in the safest manner, reducing the amount of illnesses and diseases that they have and increasing their longevity.

My Top 10 Motivators

1) Food—what we eat
2) Life changing events
3) Visualization and imaging
4) Commitment
5) Power of positive thinking
6) Mind-body connection
7) The will to live
8) Meditation
9) Yoga and chi-gung
10) Purpose

We all have different things that motivate us. Take a moment to write down 10 things that motivate you the most below.

1 _____

2 _____

3 _____

4 _____

5 _____

6 _____

7 _____

8 _____

9 _____

10 _____

DETOX FROM TELEVISION

Groucho Marx once said, "I find television very educational. Every time someone switches it on, I go into another room and read a good book." Considering that I read and write books, daily practice full-time neurosurgery, do my own stock trading on the Internet, give at least one lecture a week, am on call for neuro-surgery every seventh day and weekend, play tennis three to four days a week,

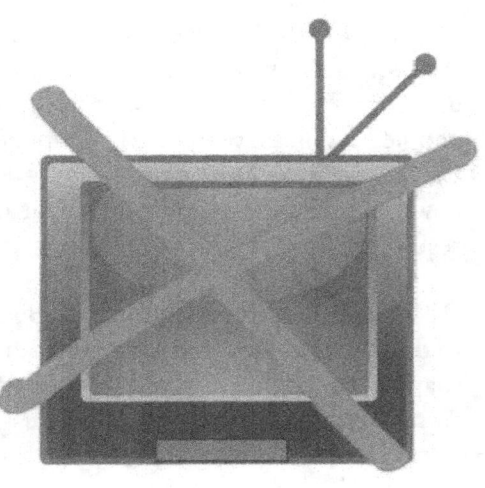

practice the piano and saxophone 20 minutes daily, take yoga lessons, it wouldn't surprise you that people asked me where I find the time. The simple answer is I get up early and don't watch TV.

I used to use TV for stress reduction, and became semi-conscious or mindless, probably a substitute for drugs or alcohol. What's interesting, I can hardly remember anything that I watched, except a few famous funerals and championship tennis matches. I gained about four hours a day saying goodbye to TV. I suggest you do the same, or perhaps you are one of the lucky few who never adopted the habit in the first place. The average American family spends seven hours a day in front of the TV. With the extra time, you can do a lot of motivating activities: join a sports club, take music lessons, read more, enjoy more time with the family in healthy activities, avoid weight gain from sitting around and snacking.

Television was invented in the 1920s, but because of World War II it did not really appear in homes much until the 1940s and 1950s. It almost instantly became hugely popular. Once television sets began appearing in homes, important changes began in the lifestyles of millions of people. Those changes have only continued and accelerated right up to the present time. Today millions of Americans watch television for as much as eight hours a day, to the point that it has become addictive behavior.

Like cigarette smoking, it is especially prevalent among the poor. Like heroin and other narcotics, it offers a fantasy world that over time can become a kind of alternate reality for the viewer. And like all addictions, it arises from the absence of genuine pleasure, joy, and fulfillment in other areas of life. TV offers an opportunity to escape the boredom of their daily lives, a desire to have something they can talk about with other people, the pleasure of seeing people advance on the screen with which they can compare the own experiences, and keeping in touch with the news and events of the world. Of course, they report mainly the bad news, resulting in bad news conversations, and nothing is said about the good things in their lives.

When there's real beauty and adventure in your life, there's no need to dramatize it by comparing yourself with characters of the sitcoms or soap operas or sports figures. When there's only boredom in your daily routine, the fabricated adventures of T.V. characters provide an alternative. An eminent psychoanalyst defined boredom as "desire for desire." We're bored when we know we want something, but we don't quite know what that something is. With a look before hand among the programs on television, we should learn to recognize our true needs and find ways to satisfy them in the things we do every day. Everyone has the ability to create genuine pleasure in his/her life. The power to create joy always remains within us, waiting to be rediscovered and explored. Turning off the television can be very motivating to a more healthy and joyful life. It sure worked for me. Learn to enjoy the experience of your own spirit, not somebody else's.

Which side of the glass do you want to live on? When you're watching television, you are watching other people do what they love doing for a living and get paid for. They are having fun and making money and you are passively watching them have fun making money. They're getting money and you're not. What do you remember, the show you watched a month ago, or the book you read and the ideas in it? The growing fascination with going online is an improvement over television, especially if you interact. Communicating inside thoughtful chat rooms and sending and receiving emails grow the brain. Certainly that can get out of hand. Television does not grow your brain; there is no cognitive stimulation, except on rare occasions

DON'T RETIRE—
KEEP A SENSE OF PURPOSE

If you stop doing things, not only your body, but your brain will also get stiff. We all have heard, use it or lose it. That is 100% true. It is also known that within five years of retirement, there is a significant death rate versus people who are still working. When you slow down too much, you come to a stop. Certainly the trick is to be working at something that you love so it's no problem to continue. Then again, some of us have had jobs that are physically very demanding, like coal mining, types of factory work, or very stressful desk jobs or dangerous jobs. But if you feel the need to retire,

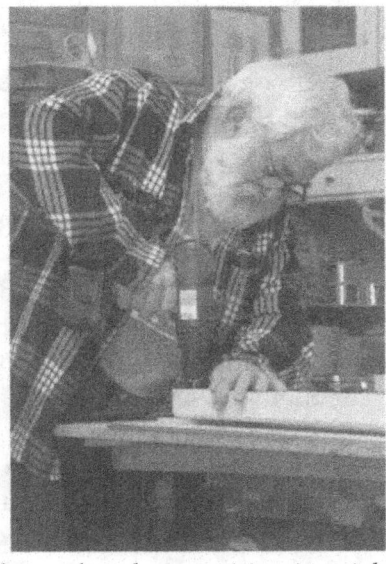

at least have a plan ready, if at all possible, so that the transition is quick and does not take a great toll on your mind.

The next job could be very simple. Like someone who carries out groceries six hours a day for four days a week. Let's face it, he's getting a lot of exercise, and is constantly talking to people of all ages and making some friends. He is very happy and healthy.

I still practice neurosurgery at age 74 and I have good results, know a lot more than the next guy because I have seen many different types of problems over my 41 years of practice. I am more experienced and have a more conservative approach compared to most surgeons. I know the body knows how to get well. I also feel I have a sense of purpose, and feel so lucky that I do. I spend a lot of time giving lectures, doing DVDs and CDs, sharing my thoughts with the public to make them well. I feel I can do at least the intellectual part of my work way into the future. I plan to be writing books when I'm 95. It is most fortunate that I have a sense of purpose. I would like you to have the same, no matter what that purpose might be. Just pour your heart and soul into it and you will live longer and keep your intelligence.

I work out regularly—yoga and weight lifting. Habits I recommend to everyone. I play tennis three to four days a week, at night, mainly. I hope to have my retirement party the day after I die. A good retirement is about one to three months.

The only people who really enjoy their retirement are those who have a purpose that substitutes totally for the time spent at work. Otherwise you will lose your sense of importance. You will spend your time at the TV watching other people while you get stiff and old, and your brain shrinks. I know many people who are just waiting to retire and travel. I spoke to one of our local politicians recently. He didn't want to run for public office again, and wanted to travel after his retirement in three years. He also had type 2 diabetes. I doubt he will be healthy enough to travel and there's a possibility he will not live that long. The prognosis for a type 2 diabetic with his abdomen hanging down is not good. Many of them have a sudden death. I know of a number of people, once they retired, within a few weeks were back at work at something else, or even the same work or business with all its problems, but they felt worth while again.

One solution to dodging full retirement is to retire partially. Work three or four days a week. It gets you out of the house, off the couch; you make some money and you meet a few people. You can always go back to college, meet some young people, learn a new language, or a new profession. Also, helping other people through volunteer work on a regular basis can also be very fulfilling, start exercising and learning some new things. Make stretching and exercise a regular part of your day. After all, if you're going to live to be a hundred, I want you to be physically and mentally strong. It can be done without that much difficulty. You just have to be persistent about it. How you think and what you do will determine the result the majority of the time. How you age will be determined by your mind.